Milestone Moments in Getting your PhD in Qualitative Research

Chandos

Information Professional Series

Series Editor: Ruth Rikowski
(email: Rikowskigr@aol.com)

Chandos' new series of books is aimed at the busy information professional. They have been specially commissioned to provide the reader with an authoritative view of current thinking.

They are designed to provide easy-to-read and (most importantly) practical coverage of topics that are of interest to librarians and other information professionals. If you would like a full listing of current and forthcoming titles, please visit www.chandospublishing.com.

New authors: we are always pleased to receive ideas for new titles; if you would like to write a book for Chandos, please contact Dr Glyn Jones on g.jones.2@elsevier.com or telephone +44 (0) 1865 843000.

Milestone Moments in Getting your PhD in Qualitative Research

Margaret Zeegers and Deirdre Barron

ELSEVIER

AMSTERDAM • BOSTON • CAMBRIDGE • HEIDELBERG
LONDON • NEW YORK • OXFORD • PARIS • SAN DIEGO
SAN FRANCISCO • SINGAPORE • SYDNEY • TOKYO
Chandos Publishing is an imprint of Elsevier

CP
CHANDOS PUBLISHING

Chandos Publishing is an imprint of Elsevier
225 Wyman Street, Waltham, MA 02451, USA
Langford Lane, Kidlington, OX5 1GB, UK

ISBN: 978-0-08-100231-5

British Library Cataloguing in Publication Data
A catalogue record for this book is available from the British Library

Library of Congress Control Number: 2015935166

For information on all Chandos Publishing
visit our website at http://store.elsevier.com/

Original cover design: Margaret Zeegers

Dedication

For my mother, Agnes Timmers, who truly understood the importance of learning. She has been a constant source of inspiration for all I have learned myself and taught others. And for my partner, Duncan, and my daughter, Elizabeth.

Zeegers

For my children, Celeste, David, Matthew, and Natalie, particularly Natalie, who is about to embark on this journey herself. And for my grandchildren, Xavier, Loki, and Aurelia.

Barron

Contents

Acknowledgments

The book has grown out of programs that we have successfully implemented in our own universities and we gratefully acknowledge all those colleagues and candidates who have contributed their expertise to make these programs successful. We are particularly grateful for those candidates who have generously allowed us to use their work for the annotated examples that appear throughout the book. In each case, they have shown just how they have themselves engaged, addressed, dealt with, and solved the sorts of problems that all research candidates face in the various milestones of their research projects. What is more, they have shown how to do so with knowledge and flair.

About the authors

Dr. Margaret Zeegers is adjunct professor within the Faculty of Health, Arts, and Design at Swinburne University of Technology, Victoria, Australia.

Dr. Deirdre Barron is associate professor in the Centre for Design Innovation, Faculty of Health, Arts, and Design, Swinburne University of Technology, Melbourne, Australia.

Introduction

The purpose of this book

This book has been written to help research candidates through the processes of undertaking and completing a PhD (or professional doctorate, masters, or honors) using qualitative research methodology and method. As there are common milestones in all qualitative research projects across all disciplines, these processes and milestones can be applied equally to any qualitative research degree which includes an individual research project undertaken in an institution that awards research-based degrees. These include course work and dissertation and Viva Voce, as in North America, and thesis production, as in Europe and British Commonwealth countries, and by publication. This last is an emerging model across all institutions, becoming increasingly prominent as more candidates opt for this. The outcomes of research undertaken in such ways share a commonality that draws on the OECD (2002) definition of research: "...Creative work undertaken on a systematic basis in order to increase the stock of knowledge, including knowledge of man [*sic*], culture and society, and the use of this stock of knowledge to devise new applications" (p. 30). Regardless of the path chosen, then, we can tease out common threads and steps to be taken for detailed consideration in communicating this knowledge generated via the written component of any research degree.

At the same time, there is a growing trend toward interdisciplinary research, leading researchers to work across discipline boundaries, such as Business and Engineering, or Education and Design. The same trend sees them combining qualitative and quantitative methods. While this trend opens up options for new and exciting ways of generating new knowledge, it still requires the same OECD outcomes. An issue for supervisors then becomes one of monitoring candidate adherence to different disciplines' expectations of research undertaken. You will read and hear of claims to mixed method, only to find that this is no more than a study that includes two or more methods, each of which needs to be dealt with appropriately as far as methodology and method requirements are concerned. The fact that a given study has statistics as well as interviews as well as document analysis, for example, does not necessarily mean mixed method; it may only mean that three methods have been used.

We have drawn on our experience of supervising and examining doctoral theses in writing this book. Given this, the programs that we have implemented, and thus this book, are based on the notion of scaffolded learning. We stress that there is a difference between the research outcome (thesis/artifact) and the processes of becoming a researcher. There is a plethora of literature on *How to write a PhD*. Such literature is most helpful but largely ignores those other factors that we have identified as part of what might be considered in the less clearly defined aspects of completing your thesis. Such things may be ways in which to start out on your research project, or administrative concerns and ways in which these may influence research outcomes. Our focus is on the processes of becoming a recognized academic researcher, which is about learning the requirements and expectations of academia. This book guides the research candidate through these processes while providing a structure that may be used to produce the thesis.

Level

The book is aimed at research candidates in that it:

- provides accessible advice and guidance across a spectrum of methodological, personal, emotional, practical, and institutional issues that are to be negotiated by an increasingly diverse student body;
- provides an account of research as methodology, method, process, and practice; and
- uses real-life experiences to demonstrate processes of thesis development.

While research inquiries are informed by rigorous theoretical and methodological principles and protocols, we have proceeded on the understanding that skill and craft progression is fundamentally developed through applying these to real-life circumstances and dilemmas. For those embarking on independent academic research, perhaps for the first time, there is huge scope for anxiety and uncertainty in applying the variety of theoretical, methodological, and technical prescriptions to their specific research activities. Each milestone addresses such candidate concerns as they apply to the various stages of the production of a thesis.

Organization

While the book is structured in such a way as to represent a typical progress toward a thesis, we stress that we do not suggest these as occurring in an orderly linear process. Your own progress in the production of the thesis may take a different order from the one suggested here. If this is the case, you will ensure that each milestone will be addressed regardless, and fit in with the timeline you have designed for your work. The order in which these milestones are engaged and reached will differ from candidate to candidate. The milestone of the literature review, for example, may be reached before or after the methodology or method milestones; the milestone of the introductory chapter may not be reached until after all the other milestones have been reached; and so on. Each milestone is dealt with separately, but each overlaps with others. Even then, several milestones may be worked toward at the same time over the years during which the thesis is produced. That is, certain targets will be achieved within the timeframe allowed, and not just in the final year.

How to use this book

While the book suggests a sequential order, and may be read in this sequence, there is nothing to preclude a reader dipping into and out of it as each milestone comes into focus. Readers are advised to focus on one milestone at a time, in the order in which they apply to their own program of studies. We recognize the role of learning within PhD (or professional doctorate or masters or honors) research to facilitate making informed choices and engagement with a range of research experiences and situations, and we have included examples from candidates to show how they have managed the processes concerned, how they have made strategic choices, and how they have developed their skills. The annotated examples given may be used by the reader as models for their own writing. The book, then, describes learning and research in practice, and the reader may embrace that learning as they proceed.

Part One

Establishing the basis for the PhD

Milestone 1: Clearing the decks

1

We come to the idea of doing a PhD through a variety of ways. For some of us, it is purely opportunistic, in getting a good Honors degree outcome, for example, and taking a further step in enrolling in a PhD. Others of us, particularly professionals in a given field, may have been thinking for some time about doing that degree. And for some of us, possibly lower order academics, the idea is thrust upon us and we have had to be talked into it. The idea has its appeal, but it does seem like an enormous undertaking, a bit like starting out on the Great Wall of China in the middle of the Gobi Desert, with Beijing a long way off, and far too many steps to take before getting there. It may seem like this, but it is not. There is a given number of milestones to reach, and each one takes you closer to your destination. What is involved in getting any Higher Degree by Research (HDR), like the Professional Doctorate and the Masters, is very similar to getting a PhD. If you are enrolled in the Masters by Research, Professional Doctorate, or Doctor of Philosophy (PhD) program then you are considered a Higher Degree Research candidate. In some countries, governments refer to their universities' Higher Degree Research programs as Research Training Degrees, or Research Training Schemes, so the terms may be used interchangeably. It is a matter of tradition that students enrolled in a HDR are referred to as a candidate. Because of the similarities involved in achieving any HDR, we will use the milestones toward achieving a PhD to identify and illustrate the milestones toward achieving one.

Reasons for not doing your PhD

You may have more reasons for NOT doing this PhD than you have for doing one, and we will start by addressing these.

Reason 1: "I will be (insert appropriate age here: 37, 42, 58, 60) years old by the time I finish."
Spoiler 1: You will be that age whether you have a PhD or not. Better to get to that age with a PhD than without one.
Reason 2: "It will take years to complete."
Spoiler 2: Of course it will. Your first degree probably took 3 or 4 years, and you managed that all right. Remember how quickly those years went by though. Your PhD will take 3 years, with a possible extension up to 4 years full time or the equivalent of this part time. The time allowed is not negotiable; there is a set duration of a Higher Degree by Research candidature. Your university is accredited and funded on completion rates and times. The normal period of candidature for doctoral candidates is 3 years, in some cases 4, and for masters' candidates 2 or 3 years. But it is not like when you were 12 and had to wait a whole year before you could be 13, an interminable age at that time. Now that you are grown up, you have yourself been despairing of the swiftness of the years going past. The time taken doing your PhD will pass just as swiftly, perhaps even more swiftly than you would like.

In our experience as supervisors, we have found that people who follow the steps that we outline and write at the rate that we suggest complete within 3 years.
Reason 3: "I haven't the time."
Spoiler 3: Nobody does. We are all adults with adult responsibilities: mortgages or rent, work, shopping, cooking, cleaning, hobbies, sport, recreation, recalcitrant partners, spoiled children, demanding in-laws, aged parents, eccentric aunts and uncles, community involvement...and this is the list for only ONE person. With parents no longer organizing our lives to free us up for studies as they did when we were at school, we take on all the responsibility ourselves. But you had that with your first degree, so you have some experience in this.
Reason 4: "I'm not smart enough."
Spoiler 4: Not so. If you can get through Grade 4 at primary school, you can get through your PhD. There is no magic or mystery involved. There are conventions to be observed, regulations to be complied with, specific tasks to be done, and that's it. You take it Milestone by Milestone, with some overlap, until you finish. What helps many of us through the PhD process is looking around us at the obvious dopes that do have their PhDs, and knowing that we are at least as smart, if not smarter, than they.
Reason 5: "I resent having to do a PhD when my years of experience, and my breadth and depth of knowledge, enable me to do my job exceptionally well."
Spoiler 5: Resent it as much as you like, but this will not help you when it comes to the jobs that are available to you at your current level of education, or promotions that stipulate that a PhD or substantial progress toward getting one as a requirement of the position. We would also point out that practical knowledge, valuable as it is, is not the same as the knowledge generated by research. A teacher who develops and implements excellent programs for their students, who then achieve excellent outcomes, is no doubt a great teacher. They are not considered education researchers, though.
Reason 6: "I object to the creeping credentialism of my workplace and absolutely refuse to submit to this."
Spoiler 6: So who are you hurting by taking this stance? Your own silent protest is quite ineffectual and does not do a thing to prevent the creeping at all. You are the only one being adversely affected. The creeping credentialism that put a stop to butcher surgeons and hairdresser dentists has been a boon to us all, not a disadvantage.
Reason 7: "I do all right as I am. I got jobs ahead of others more qualified than I and have gone ahead faster than just about everybody else."
Spoiler 7: That's wonderful for you, but you are going to hit a brick wall any day now because there is a point beyond which you cannot proceed until you get your PhD. You will watch those others that you passed on your way up, who knuckled down and did their PhDs, now start passing you on their onward and upward journeys. At the same time, though, if you do not need it and do not want it, don't do it. You need read no further.
Reason 8: "Everybody else has already researched my field. I have nothing that I could add."
Spoiler 8: That's not what a PhD is about. You are not going to be covering a whole field, but a part of it. People may have written an awful lot about things that are important in your field, but not in relation to your particular position within that field. There are things that may have been overlooked, and what you have in mind may present a different perspective that may challenge, enhance, or expand accepted knowledge within that field.
Reason 9: "I hated my major studies in my first degree. The last thing I want to do is get involved with that stuff again."
Spoiler 9: If this is so, look for areas within that field that are more interesting and worthy of further exploration. A PhD is a way to cross fields. You may have studied Economics the first time around, and use this to study the position of the anonymous and unnamed servants

in Jane Austen's books. Whether you decide to research in the area in which you want to work, or you take up a position within an established research project that interests you, you may make your own decisions about where you want your PhD to take you.

Reason 10: "I can't afford it."

Spoiler 10: If we all took that approach, we would have no education at all. It is always expensive, because it is so valuable. The government of your country recognizes the importance of postgraduate studies and their timely completions, and will have policy in place to encourage postgraduate studies. This policy may include student loans, scholarship provision, waived fees, student stipends, or a combination of these developed to optimize the likely successful completion of a candidate's program of study, support the development of graduate attributes as specified by governments and taken up by universities, and comply with government requirements in general.

You will probably find that your local university is rather keen to take on PhD candidates to benefit its own standing in the research community and with its funding bodies and will have its plans in place to attract such candidates. They may waive the tuition fees, offer part or full scholarships, and so on. Where your country's government offers scholarships, there will be published criteria and guidelines for applying for these, so it is worthwhile investigating them, and positioning yourself according to the published criteria. Your university of preference may offer its own forms of scholarships, with application dates at various times of the year, and you may also position yourself for one of these: Do they have points system, for example, for progress in studies, an Honors or Masters degree (or both), a number of publications in scholarly and professional journals? Or something different: practice in the field, consultancies, advisory committee work? Or a combination of these? Be familiar with the requirements, and work towards meeting the requirements (by having work published and so on) before the closing date.

You could probably come up with more reasons, indeed you might already have, and they would be quite reasonable in your circumstances. It is also probable that you could come up with spoilers yourself and give yourself very good reasons for going ahead with your PhD. Going ahead with it means taking up the idea of research and its contribution to knowledge.

What research is

At the very start, you need to come to terms with just what this sort of degree is. It is called an HDR because it is based on research. The Shorter Oxford English Dictionary (OED) defines research as an "endeavour to discover new or collate old facts etc. by scientific study of a subject, [or] course of critical investigation." People who call themselves researchers actually do what is recognized by their peers as research. Research is also any means by which a discipline or art develops, tests, and renews itself. All of these meanings are complementary (and overlap) and all have a place in universities.

Yet another way of thinking about what research means is to consider the different ways in which those who do it might identify a given activity as research. There are three common ways in which communities of researchers see the work they call research as being distinctive: it adopts a characteristic theoretical perspective; it pursues a characteristic central question or problem; or it adopts a characteristic method. Research, then, as the Organisation for Economic Cooperation and Development (OECD) (2002) says, is generating new knowledge or using existing knowledge in new ways (which is generating new knowledge anyway). Most of us take the second route, working with what others before us have done and developing, extending, or building on that. Research is not simply reading everything that everybody else has written on the subject and reproducing it. It is examining what everybody else has written on the subject and showing how what you have found contributes to what other people have already done. This requires original research on your part, investigating aspects of a subject that are still to be engaged in your field. What results will be your reinterpretation of existing knowledge and contributing new knowledge of your own in the process of your research.

What your thesis is

Then you need to come to terms with the fact that you are writing a thesis, not a book, and that you are writing it for your two or three examiners, not your supervisor(s) or the general public. You need to engage the idea of genre here. A genre as far as we are concerned here is a text type. Each text type or genre has its own particular characteristics, characteristics that each reader and writer may expect to see in the text. We have the genre of novels, text books, short stories, poems, reports, newspaper articles, scholarly articles, scholarly books, and so on. The thesis is a particular genre of its own, and every chapter is another one of these genres, a subgenre of the thesis genre (see "Milestone 10: Drawing conclusions and making recommendations" chapter). You probably have never written in this genre before, and you probably never will again, but this does not mean that it cannot be learned. You will find that when you are supervising your own PhD candidates, which you will be expected to do as a qualified academic in a university, you will help them to learn it as well.

You have had to learn to write in other genres, such as the academic essay, the research report, the formal letter, perhaps poetry and creative narrative. In each case, you learned that there are specific features of the genre to be considered and applied. You can learn it for a thesis as well. The important thing is not to write it in the same way as the scholarly books, chapters, and articles that you will consult as your study proceeds, but as a thesis that will be examined by research experts in your field. Even so, this whole process has the added dimension of becoming a researcher and becoming doctorly yourself. It is part of the training in research that leads you to position yourself as a recognized researcher in your field, becoming one of those experts yourself.

Putting the proposal together

Once you have decided that you are going to do a PhD, it is time to establish just what you will be researching, in what ways, and with whom. You will think these things through and you will put a proposal together for submission to the university of your choice. You will give a title (which will probably change by the time that you submit) and provide a

250-word summary of your proposed research. Your chosen university will have an administrative department for its research and research student activities, such as a Graduate School, or a Research and Graduate Office, or some such thing. They will take it from there, assessing your application, canvassing appropriate supervisors, and so on.

Getting the question

One of the first things to consider for your PhD proposal is what you will be researching, so you will formulate a research question. Note that the word, *question*, is what is used here. It is not *problem* or *issue*. Problems and issues may be covered in things like research reports, which are a different genre from that of thesis. What is more, the sort of question that you will formulate will be a *how* or *why* question. It will not be a *what* question (again, this is the sort of question dealt with in research reports). Remember your definition of research: generating new knowledge or using existing knowledge in new ways. *What* will only take you to the existing knowledge. It will not take you into the realms of *generating* new knowledge or *using* existing knowledge *in new ways*.

There is a history of approaches to research in all disciplines that address questions of a practical or technical kind. In education, for example, we perennially address the problem of what should be taught and learned; the museum sciences continually focus on technical questions of how natural and cultural artifacts can best be conserved and preserved. Some of these questions are philosophical (or conceptual or speculative, or both) and are explicitly focused on normative questions rather than empirical ones. You will focus on such questions, and not even consider things like hypotheses to be tested, or any truth to be established, or any beliefs you might hold being tested. In our type of research, qualitative research, we do not work with a hypothesis, we seriously question the notion of truth, refuse to entertain the idea of reality, and find that belief is just not good enough for a researcher to go on.

Concepts to be engaged

You will work with established concepts, though. One of the first to get your head around is that of theory and the role that this plays in your research.

Theory

This is what will be the basis of your research. Because your question is not a *what happens when…* but a *why or how does it happen when…* sort of question, you will draw on a theory to explain the *why* or the *how*. The word *theory* and the concept of theory itself have very specific meanings to the researcher. A theory is not a hypothesis, or something to be proved or established, for that has already been done by researchers before you came on the scene. It is not speculation; it is not an informed guess or a hunch. It is a set of principles or statements based on evidence, and accepted by the research field. In research terms, a theory may be shown to apply across all situations for a theory is a set of principles that has been shown to explain, and been generally accepted as, why or how something happens. You might hear people being dismissive of something, like Darwin's theory of evolution, saying something like, "But it's only a theory" (Fry, 2013). A theory is not an insignificant *only* at all as far as research is concerned; it is the result of careful research to establish the acceptability of certain knowledge. Because of its general acceptance within a research field, a theory may be applied to other phenomena to explain them as well. In general conversation, we might say something like, "I have a theory about people being cat rather than dog people," and there is no problem with that in that context. In this case, we are speculating and hypothesizing, which is what people do in everyday life.

In a research project, this will not do; it does not hold for us as researchers because a theory, in a research sense, is not under question. We need an accepted and established theory about which there is no question. This applies to positivist and quantitative research—the theory of gravity, or subatomic theory—and to interpretivist and qualitative research, such a poststructuralism or phenomenology or symbolic interactionism. In the research world in which you are working, a theory is a generally accepted explanation for something happening. There are many theories from which you may select. This does not mean that one theory is better than another; it just means that one is more suitable to your research needs than any other.

In your research, the theory with which you work is your **methodology**. Your methodology is a theory of producing knowledge through research and provides a rationale for the way you will proceed as a researcher. It underpins your research.

Data

This is always plural (*the data show/indicate/suggest*). It is the raw material that you generate in your research. Your data may be the responses to interviews, questionnaires, surveys, the wording or phrasing of documents, the items in diaries or journals, your observation notes, photographs, video tapes, audio tapes, transcripts of interviews, and so on. You may have the figures of the numbers of horses, troops, and ships brought by William the Conqueror to England, but this is data only. It remains data until you analyze it in relation to the theory that you have selected to underpin your research. Data are very much part of your concern as a researcher, but until you do your analytical work with them, that is all that they are.

Information

This is what your data become as part of your analysis. It is the facts of what you have encountered in your research. Information is facts, figures, and so on that you have gleaned from your data. Information of and by itself is never knowledge; it is yet to be filtered through your theory and applied as a meaningful thing if it is to become knowledge. As information, it is a very public thing that has not been internalized. You know that the year 1066 is the date of the King Richard's losing the Battle of Hastings to William the Conqueror, but it is no more than information until you do something with it. While information will feature in your research project, it is not the major consideration for you as a researcher. Knowledge is, though.

Knowledge

Knowledge is when information and data are filtered through experience and applied as a meaningful thing. When you put the year 1066 together with the numbers of horses, troops, and boats brought by William the Conqueror to England and use this to engage historical interpretations of the import of the King Richard's loss of the Battle in wreaking enormous social, political, and economic change in England at the time, then you are in the realm of knowledge. You will address the data and information that you generate in relation to the theory that you are using, and in doing so you will generate the knowledge that is integral to your PhD activities.

Positioning yourself as the researcher

As you read qualitative research publications, such as scholarly books, chapters in scholarly books, articles in research journals, and conference proceedings, you will notice that in some cases the author or authors refer to themselves as *the researcher* or *the researchers*, following this up with passive voice expressions: *it was established that...*; *it was observed that...;* and other such phrasing. They have done this as they have taken on board suggestions of objectivity in their research being reflected in such language use. Others will refer to themselves in the first person (*I, me, we, us, my, our*) and use active voice in their phrasing: *I/we established that*...; *we observed that....* These researchers have rejected the notion that such language use suggests objectivity, indeed insisting on making it apparent that there is a certain subjectivity to be taken on board in qualitative research in interpretivist traditions.

You will make decisions regarding this sort of thing when you present your own research in your thesis or other forms of research writing. It is a decision based on more than personal preference or academic style. It is a decision based on ways in which you see yourself as a researcher. We take the position that the first person pronoun and active voice be used, for we are qualitative researchers and we do not attempt to hide or camouflage the subjectivity that we have indeed embraced in our activities as researchers. Scheurich (1997), in his discussions on issues of validity in qualitative research, is instructive on this point. As you achieve more milestones down the track, you would be advised to read this work closely for you may be asked to put a scholarly argument for first person and active voice in your writing, but at this point it is enough that you make the decision regarding ways in which you will position yourself when you write up your own research (see also "Milestone 2: The confirmation or defence of candidature" chapter).

Negotiating the supervisor

Unless you have already approached an experienced and active researcher prepared to supervise you upon acceptance of your proposal, the university will make approaches on your behalf. They know who is working in what fields, the expertise they have, their track record of timely completions by candidates, and so on. The coordinating or principal supervisor is required to be experienced in postgraduate supervision and to be an active researcher with expertise in the candidate's field. They are responsible for ensuring that each candidate's research is conducted ethically and appropriately for the field and methodology concerned, and assisting candidates to present their project in a form worthy of examination for the degree. The associate supervisor is usually someone who can contribute to the candidates' postgraduate studies through their research experience. A candidate may have other supervisors appointed to their team where that supervisor brings important expertise to the supervisory team (as in panels). At the very least, you will have a Principal Supervisor, who will take up major responsibilities on your behalf, and an Associate Supervisor, who will also play an important role in supervising your studies.

In the traditional model of supervision your coordinating supervisor will normally be the person who undertakes the majority of the supervision of your research project. You can expect your coordinating supervisor to offer advice on the focus of your research, the methodology that will underpin your project, and the method you will employ to carry out the research. Your coordinating supervisor should also provide guidance on the development and presentation of your research outcomes, for faculty seminars, conferences, and publication as well as the examinable outcome. You will organize regular meetings with your supervisors and in particular with your principal or coordinating supervisor. Note that it is you who will do this, not your supervisor.

In the panel model of supervision, the panel chair will normally be responsible for oversight of the administrative details of your progress and for ensuring that each of the panel members is providing appropriate advice to your project. You will ensure that you know which panel member will provide advice on methodology, method, and presentation. You will establish a calendar of meeting times with panel members and the panel as a whole.

Given the emerging trend for cross-disciplinary and multiple methods research, the supervisory team or panel can be expected to comprise experts from different disciplines. In this situation, the need for detailed and careful communication regarding the requirements of the research features of each discipline cannot be underestimated. As always, good communication will align the various positions that supervisors from different disciplines may bring to a supervisory team.

Note that they are called *supervisors*, not teachers, lecturers, tutors, or other such words that might suggest that they are the source of knowledge or responsible for your progress in your studies. You are the person who will be generating that knowledge, and they are there to guide in doing so in accordance with protocols, regulations, conventions, and ethics. Supervising and guiding is not the same as teaching and tutoring, and your studies are essentially your own responsibility under that supervision and guidance as you progress as an independent researcher.

There are several options to be taken up here. If you are enrolled on the basis of being included in an existing project being conducted by a team of researchers, the leader of that project will be your Principal Supervisor, and other experienced and qualified people working on that project will be your Associate Supervisors. If you are working on a research project by yourself, your Principal Supervisor and an Associate Supervisor will work with you. Note the word is *with*; it is not *for*.

In Australia, the Deans and Directors of Graduate Studies (DDoGS) (Council of Australian Deans and Directors of Graduate Studies, 2005) provide an indication of the role of the supervisor(s), especially the principal supervisor, who "has a significant role in the development of discipline specific research skills and more general skills such as those relating to information and technological literacies, ethics, IP (Intellectual Property), scholarly publishing, conference presentations, etc." Universities proceed on the basis of this sort of indications from appropriate bodies in the countries concerned. The policies of your university will reflect this sort of general statement on the role of the supervisor(s).

You and your supervisor(s) will be advised by the university to negotiate the protocols for working together: the frequency of meetings; submission of and feedback on drafts of chapters; the ways that you will (or will not) publish together from out of your research; the reaching of the various milestones and the timeframes for these; the means by which you will communicate be that by things such e-mail, phone, Skype, face-to-face, or a combination of these; the timing and completion of progress reports on your studies; ethics application and issues associated with this; and so on. Such things are best established at the outset, so that both parties have clear expectations of each other.

The words used

You are now coming to terms with your PhD having two parts to it.

- The first is the research itself, conducted according to established rules and conventions of research. The second is the thesis in which this research is reported, again in accordance with established rules and conventions of thesis production. The thesis is what you submit for examination. Doing your PhD is essentially undergoing a 3- to 4-year examination (or part time equivalent). You will be quite clear in your use of the words, *research* and *thesis*, not using them interchangeably.
- You will frame your research around *how* and *why* questions, resisting the temptation to include any that begin with *what*.
- You will focus on the formulation of research questions, and forget all about any notions that you might have had about hypotheses, for these do not belong in qualitative research.
- You will distinguish between data, information, and knowledge, not using these interchangeably.

Suggested reading

Blaikie, N. (1993). *Approaches to social enquiry* is similar to Flick's work, a good summary of research issues.

Flick, U. (2007). *Designing qualitative research* may be helpful when working towards the next milestone, the Confirmation of Candidature.

Flick, U. (2009). *An introduction to qualitative research* especially useful in its accessible language and clarity of concepts.

Conclusion

None of this is more than you can handle. Many, many of your peers have their PhDs, after all, and you can get one as well. The next milestone that you will take up is the Confirmation of Candidature, due in about a year (or the equivalent part time). Despite any perceived problems you might have in the early stages, there is a lot to be said for having a PhD, and very little against.

Hot Tip 1

Set up your Headings for chapters and their subheadings using the Styles function on your computer, and use them from the very start of writing your thesis when you come to submit it for examination. Headings through Styles means a click of a button to compile your Table of Contents, List of Tables, and List of Figures. This will save you hours, possibly weeks, of work with your Confirmation of Candidature document in the first instance, as well as the thesis later.

Milestone 2: The confirmation or defense of candidature

2

In most universities, once you are accepted as a PhD candidate (which what you will be called until you submit), you will have the equivalent of a year's full-time study to prepare your Confirmation of Candidature (sometimes also called the Colloquium). In some universities, what is required is some sort of oral defense of your project (sometimes called the Viva Voce, or Viva for short). The panel that is convened for this process need not all necessarily be from your field, but you will be told who they are and this will give you some idea of their backgrounds. Some of them will be experts in research itself…ways of designing and conducting research in general…not necessarily in designing and conducting research in your area specifically. If it is done toward the beginning of your research program, you will convince them, on the basis of what you have written and what you have to say in your oral presentation and their questioning of you, that you have in effect emerged from that initial 12-month probationary period because you have shown not only that you have developed a viable PhD research program and have made satisfactory progress over the previous 12 months, but also that you will be able to submit in a timely fashion. If it occurs after you have completed your research, you will convince them, on the basis of what you have written and what you have to say in your presentation and in response to their questioning of you, that you have indeed met all the demands of a successful PhD research program. Your thesis is the document that forms the basis of this process. We will proceed on the basis of a Confirmation of Candidature or Colloquium occurring toward the beginning of the research undertaking, generally within the first year of candidature. See "Milestone 11: Finishing, submitting, and examination" chapter which looks at Viva Voce in more detail.

The panel of experts will look at your work very seriously and provide carefully considered advice on the basis of their engagement with your work. Because the focus is on the feasibility of the research you have proposed, the structure of the panel of experts comes from a range of research fields. They will know your work as well as you will enable them to know it. It is in your hands; you will write a document that details what you propose to do.

Designing the research

There are certain elements to consider in producing the document, whether it is the Confirmation of Candidature or Colloquium document, or the thesis itself. The following diagram gives an indication of how you might proceed. You will find in your reading of the literature on the conduct of research that scholars do not always agree on whether something is to be considered methodology or method, and indeed that some scholars conflate the two as if they mean the same thing. You will find that they refer to a technique as a method, or that they insist that what has been called a method is really a methodology. Our advice is not to engage in this sort of debate in your writing of your thesis, for it may become a rather messy line of argument to pursue. It is not necessary for you to try to resolve academic differences about such things in your thesis. We suggest that you leave that sort of discussion to those who have already made their names as researchers and writers about research, and focus on presenting your own research in such a way as to convince your examiner(s) that you have successfully engaged in trustworthy research in accordance with established conventions. We suggest that you work with concepts of paradigm, methodology, method, and technique as separate concepts, showing that you have consulted the most relevant literature on each of these, and not conflate them or use them interchangeably. What you will be aiming for is consistency in your use of these terms throughout your document.

Given this, you proceed on the basis of the paradigm that guides you in designing the research that you will do. The paradigm guides you in decisions that you make in relation to your research, serving to establish your research position. Once you have positioned your research in relation to a given paradigm, a number of other decisions follow in a logical manner, as suggested in the diagram (Figure 1).

This is so much more than that 250-word summary of your research that you provided upon application. You will present an overview of the design of the research that will form the basis for its actual conduct and the writing of the thesis. As you do this, your supervisors will work through it with you, and your university will provide guidelines for what you are to write and what you will present orally. You will do a lot of the groundwork for your final thesis here. Much of what you cover here will form the basis of that final thesis, with the difference being that in this document you write it in future tense: "I will study…," "I will interview…," "I will analyse…," and so on. You will change to present tenses, such as present perfect tense, for the thesis itself: "I have studied…," "I have interviewed…," "I have analysed…."

We can tease out the various elements for the creation of this document. There are specific terms to be used in relation to each, providing you with the opportunity to explore, discuss, and debate as you engage scholarly discussions of them. When we use the term, *scholarly*, we mean that you will draw on the literature that you consult, to explain to the panel members (and later the examiners of your thesis) just how well you understand these concepts and the research literature that surrounds them.

These elements will be extended and expanded further in more detailed discussions about writing the various chapters of your thesis (see Part Two). A real advantage of the Confirmation of Candidature is that from the outset of your PhD you get the various elements and ways in which they are to be addressed in your head. Each element is considered in more detail below.

Paradigm

The easiest way to approach the idea of a paradigm is to see it as a sort of model that might be followed when conducting research. A paradigm is a package of attitudes and methods tied together to inform the conduct of research. It provides a conceptual

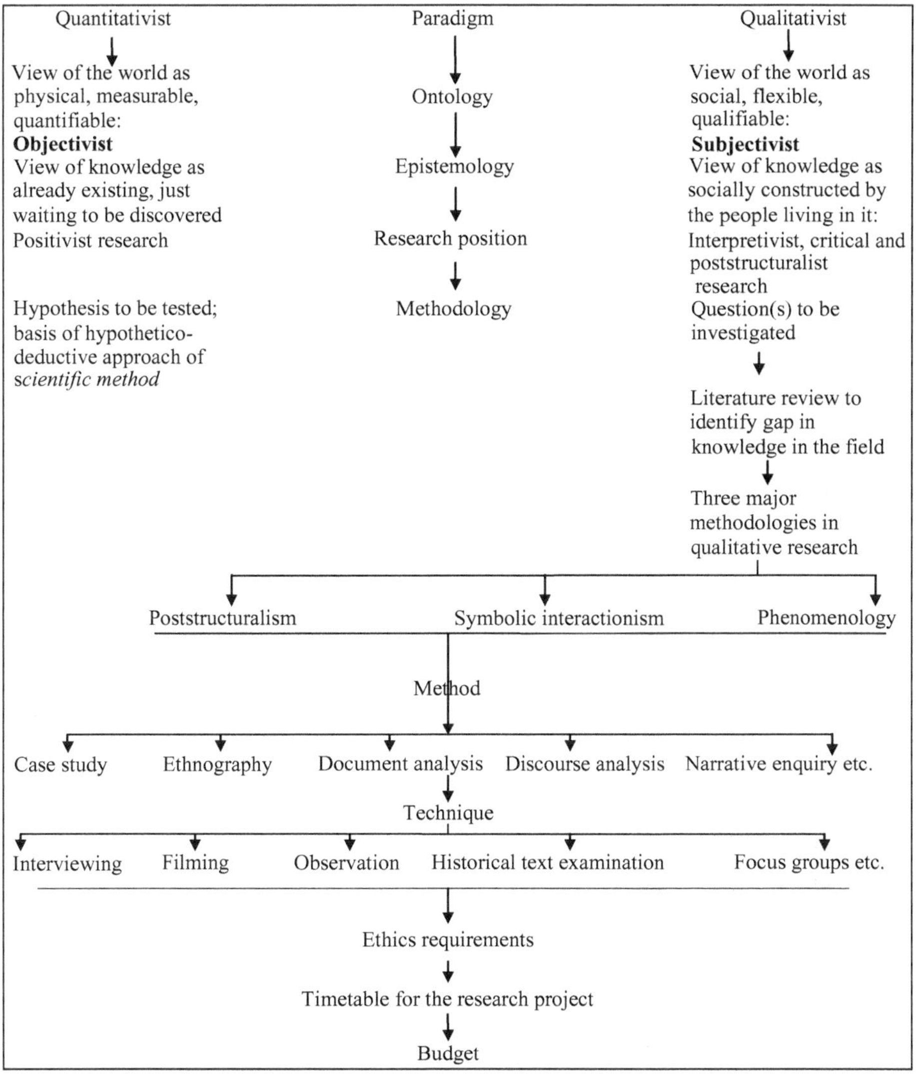

Figure 1 Framework for research.

framework to use when designing your research. A positivist will use a different paradigm from one used by an interpretivist. A positivist will not have the same ends in mind as an interpretivist in relation to paradigm, for they will be seeking to uncover truth and facts as quantitatively specified relations among variables. They will also be aiming for predictions and explanations of their physical world, claiming research rigor, internal and external validity, and reliability, in a linear process of hypothesis statement, experimentation, and quantifiable and measureable conclusion(s). For these reasons, they will work with hypothesis and all things associated with these, a hypothetico-deductive paradigm that they call *scientific method.* You will not get involved in this sort of thing. You will be using an *interpretivist* paradigm.

An interpretivist will describe meanings, seek to understand participants' definitions of the situation(s) in which they find themselves, and examine ways in which subjective realities are produced. They will aim for trustworthiness and authenticity in relation to the conclusions they make, and they will work with research questions to be investigated and all things associated with these. You will engage qualitative research, using a different, appropriate paradigm for this type of research.

Qualitative researcher

As a qualitative researcher, you will not only acknowledge subjectivity but see it as essential to the success of your research as you will not try to establish absolutes. Qualitative research is descriptive, subjective, conducted in social settings, and interpreted in relation to meanings generated by people to capture perceptions, experiences, and values. Qualitative researchers will conduct investigations *with participants,* not *on subjects,* using participant observation, interviews, conversations, diaries, journals, documents, and so on as these address aspects of social, cultural, political, and economic features of human life. You will have started out with a research question, but as you have proceeded you will probably have found that there are subsidiary questions to address as well. Your Confirmation of Candidature document will then state your Principal Research Question and Subsidiary Research Question(s). You will not take up the idea of a hypothesis at all.

Taking up the qualitative

When you write your Confirmation of Candidature document you will argue your case for taking up the position of a qualitative researcher, drawing on the substantial body of literature available to you to support a scholarly argument to this effect. It is not enough to state what you believe or think in this regard, for you are not yet an expert researcher, and you need to convince the panel of your understanding of this positioning of yours. Your positioning of yourself in the use of the first person pronoun and active voice tends toward a certain consistency as far as your being a qualitative researcher within interpretivist traditions is concerned. Given this, you will write things like: "I will conduct a series of interviews with participants to examine ways in which they negotiate social dimensions of their professional lives." You will NOT write things like: "A series of interviews with subjects on their negotiations of social dimensions of professional lives will be conducted by the researcher." You will acknowledge the subjectivity of your position, and not pretend that you do not exist by referring to yourself as *the researcher*, and you will not use the passive voice of *will be conducted by* (see the "Milestone 5: Methodology" chapter for a more detailed discussion of ways in which you position yourself as a researcher).

Literature review

You will constantly refer to your reading when you write the various sections of your document, but there is a particular section that is called the Literature Review that looks at a particular type of literature. This is the literature of published research in the field you are studying. You will engage this literature, examining the work of others in your field, noting what they have found out already, and what they are yet to find out. It is in the area of what is still to be found out that you will be working, and you will identify this as a gap in the literature on research in your field that you will address in your own research. It is not the same literature that you will engage on things like methodology, method, and technique, which deals generally and specifically with what research means and how it may be designed and carried out. The literature on which your literature review is based is on actual research that has been undertaken or is being undertaken in your field. At the Confirmation of Candidature stage, you will have done a great deal of reading, certainly, but compared with what you will have done by the time you get to thesis itself you are only just starting to make a dent in it. You will review this literature because you need to convince the panel that there really is a need for the research that you propose, given the gap in existing knowledge in the field under your consideration that you have identified. Your preliminary reading may indicate that broad brushstroke research has been published, but that there is a lack of fine-grained or detailed research in relation to specific cases in the field in general, and in your area of the field in particular. Identifying a gap in the literature is crucial, but you also need to be able to demonstrate why this gap ought to be addressed by your research. There are many gaps in many bodies of literature, after all, but this of and by itself does not indicate that research needs to be done to address those gaps. Given this, you will argue that your investigation will contribute to professional discussions and debates on a significant aspect in the field that has been the subject of some neglect. When you do this, you will be showing the significance of your research in relation identified gaps in the literature.

Methodology

Methodology is the theory of producing knowledge through research that you will use. It provides a rationale for the way you proceed a researcher. Methodology is more than particular activities, such as *doing a survey* or *interviewing people*. It answers the question of how you should go about finding out knowledge. Beginning PhD students often conflate or confuse methodology with *method*. This needs to be sorted out in your head at the outset, for *methodology* provides reasons for turning to particular *method* in relation to the kind of knowledge or understanding you are seeking. In qualitative research, we turn to three main and broad categories: poststructuralism, phenomenology, and symbolic interactionism. There are subcategories of these: critical theory, feminist theory, liberal theory, pragmatism, reconstructionism, and so on. These are the tools that you will use to inform your decisions regarding method, strategies, and data analysis in your research. You will select one of these on the basis of further reading that you will do on methodology and use it to underpin your research, in consultation with your supervisors (see the "Milestone 5: Methodology" chapter for a more detailed discussion on methodology).

Method

Method is what you use to generate the data that you will analyze, drawing on the methodology selected. It is a way of proceeding in gathering data. That data that you gather will form the basis of the knowledge that you generate through your research. Your method will proceed from the methodology you are using. You may use case study method, ethnography, narrative enquiry, and so on. Method is more on the practical side of doing research; methodology is on the theoretical (the *ology* at the end of the word tells you this) (see the "Milestone 6: Method" chapter for a more detailed discussion on method).

Validity

This is a word we come across often in relation to research, even though it is one that we do not readily take to, as the concept does not sit easily within an interpretivist paradigm and qualitative research. The concept of validity is integral to positivist research which positions knowledge in the realm of experienced, observable phenomena which can be measured and quantified. That is not the sort of research in which the interpretivist engages. Lather (1986, 1993) in suggesting the idea of *a kind of validity* to be considered, established, and maintained, has given us the concept of *trustworthiness* in relation to issues of validity in interpretative research. Scheurich (1997) says that issues of validity are *masks* which may preclude or distinguish the knowledge of the untrustworthy or the invalid from the rest. Lather and Scheurich, then, provide us with different concepts to work with when establishing the quality of our research and associated discussions of validity. These are the issues that we will discuss under a broader umbrella than *validity* alone implies (see the "Milestone 6: Method" chapter for a more detailed discussion on validity).

Technique

One could reasonably argue that all data-gathering techniques fall into one of the following three categories: listening to (or interviewing or interrogating) participants; observing behavior of participants; and examining historical or contemporary traces and records. You may use document analysis, audio taped or written interviews of research participants, field notes, diaries and journals, and a combination of each of these and indeed others.

Ethics requirements

Unless your university asks otherwise, you will generally not be required to have successfully submitted an application to whatever constitutes its mechanism for ensuring that ethics considerations have been carefully adhered to. It may be called something like the Human Research Ethics Committee (HREC). Your university may have a policy of all its researchers undergoing formal training of some sort in ethics, and you would be well advised to ensure that you have plenty of time to do this if your university requires it, well before you need to submit an ethics application. You will, though, be well advised to show in your Confirmation of Candidature document and oral presentation that you have given some serious and detailed thought to this application. You will show that you are aware of particular requirements for various groups: children participants under 18 years of age (they may be participants in research, but there are particular requirements in place for this); Indigenous or First Nation participants (there is usually a separate and particular set of requirements in these cases); people in a dependant relationship with you (you might be the one who marks their assessment tasks, for example, so they may not feel that they are able to decline; you might be their boss or line manager; they may have a family relationship with you); and so on. The fact that a dependent relationship exists does not necessarily mean that you cannot do the research with them as participants; it means that you have to put particular safeguards in place and ensure that these are complied with. You need to show that you are aware of such things, and that you have taken them into consideration (see the "Milestone 3: Getting ethics clearance" chapter for a more detailed discussion on ethics).

Timetable

You will set out a plan for completing your research, writing your thesis, and submitting it for examination. Below is an example done by a candidate who is completing their PhD part-time.

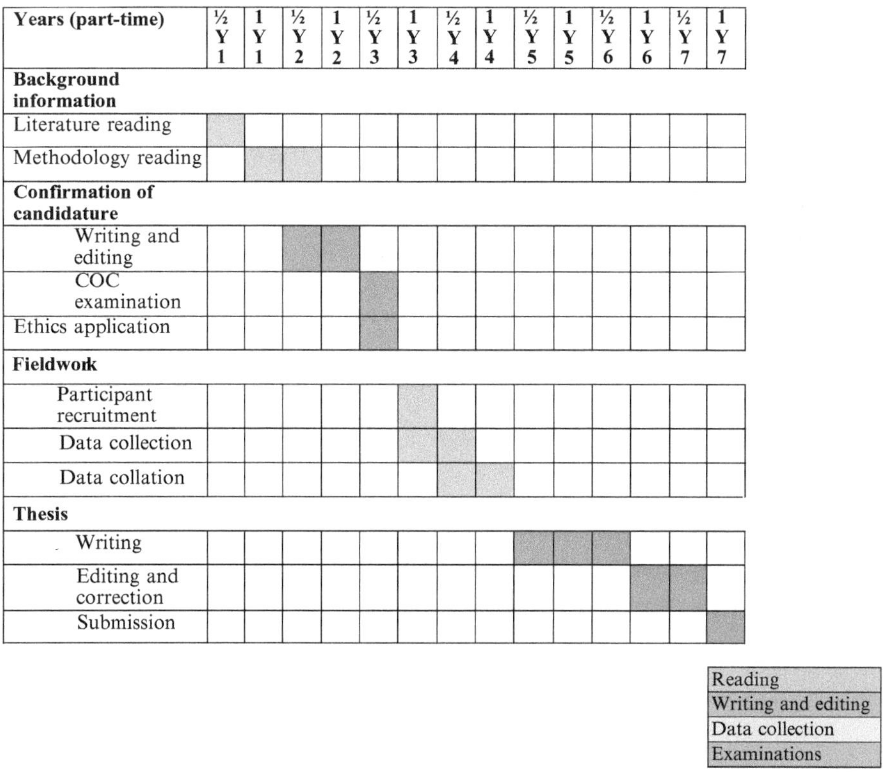

Figure 2 Research project timetable.

Budget

The exercise of confirmation is also designed to show that you understand what it means to be a researcher at this level. Part of this is to understand that all research has some cost involved, even if it is only for the time that you will take to do certain things (such as so many hours at so many dollars per hour). You may need to consider travel expenses to get to your research sites, costs of transcription services, or translation services, or license fees for specialized software for the type of research you are going to be doing. You may need to travel to conferences, and there are costs of registration, travel, meals, and accommodation to be considered. Even if your research is unfunded, the panel will expect that you show that you understand that there are costs involved (such as your time, costs of hardware and software, interview equipment hired or purchased, fuel costs for traveling to sites, costs for communicating by telephone, and/or electronic means, and so on). The panel needs to know the costs involved and how you have calculated them, whether they are privately funded (by you) or not. And even if you do not anticipate anything much in the way of spending, the panel will expect you to have taken what little will be expended into account. Most universities provide nominal funding to PhD candidates, so you may be able to design your budget around this amount, plus private sources if this is required, and present a budget as part of your research design.

Oral presentation

Your presentation is entirely under your own control. The one thing that you cannot control is the questions that the panel members may put to you. Spend some time identifying the areas in your proposal that might attract questions. These are usually around methodology and method, but you may be thrown by an unanticipated one on an area that you have not focused on so much, such as aspects of ethics that you may not have considered as carefully as you might have done. Rehearsal will help with this. So will a little background reading on the scholarly work of various panel members, whose names will be given to you, to give you an idea of their research interests.

The oral presentation presents you with an opportunity to demonstrate that your research is of the required good quality within your field. Your presentation is not an ancillary aspect of the Confirmation of Candidature; it is an integral element of it. You will have produced a pithy summary of the larger document and speak to it in a knowledgeable way, and you have been able to do this because you have done all the work required with some depth and detail. Your oral presentation is not at all the same as the written work, and it is of considerable benefit to you as a researcher as you will be able to test out your research thinking with a live audience and receive responses. It is here that you will demonstrate your developing doctoral standing, as an articulate and knowledgeable candidate. You will dress the part, you will talk the part, and you will act the part, adhering strictly to the guidelines that you have been given. You will not run over time, and you will be prepared for questions from the panel. Your principal supervisor may be of some assistance while you are being questioned, but the supervisor's role is a restricted one. Given your understanding of current debates in the field, and your background reading on panel members, you will try to anticipate the sorts of questions you might be asked during this part of the proceedings.

It is an important part of your training. You will be required, over the course of your career, to deliver oral presentations to both academic and public audiences, such as when you present your research papers at conferences. It is an integral element in defending your own methodological positioning and responding to critical questions about how you conduct your research. You would be well advised to embrace the opportunity and make the most of it. It is not something to be dreaded. It is quite a thing to have so many experts in the field, who will be your peers when you complete your PhD, taking your work so seriously.

Support groups

A PhD can be a solitary pursuit, but it need not be a lonely one. Get involved with your university's Post Graduate Student Association, its individual Schools' and Faculties' research student groups, and attend the research student activities workshops and social activities.

You would also be well advised to rehearse your presentation in front of such a group, which constitutes a knowledgeable audience, and your supervisor(s). Such a rehearsal will help you in anticipating possible questions from the panel and give you a chance to prepare appropriate answers.

The words used

For the research question itself, the words that you will use are *in what ways do*, *why do/does*, and so on. Avoid the *what* question at all costs, but where you want to refer to what already exists, write something like, *As part of my investigation, I will map the field of existing research....*

- The words that you will use in relation to your activities are those like *examine, explore*, and *investigate* the *research question(s).* You will not *prove*, *verify*, or *test* a *hypothesis,* and you will not be looking to establish *truth.*
- When you give an account of the literature that you have engaged so far, you will say something like, *My preliminary review of the literature suggests/indicates.*
- You use the standard types of phrasing for reasons that you propose this research: *I anticipate that my research will contribute to professional debates and discussions on...*
- When you discuss methodology, you will refer to this as *theoretical tools to inform my research, the theoretical underpinning of my research*, and so on. You will not refer to methodology as a framework, for this is not a function of methodology.
- You will say that you will *draw on* particular authors, ideas, or works.
- As will be writing a scholarly work, you will be working with evidence to support any claims that you make. This evidence is that which is reported in the literature.

Words not to be used

- You will not say that you *agree with* any particular authors, ideas, or works, for you do not have the authority (yet) to make such declarations. In any case, whether you agree or not has no place in research. You are to work with data and evidence. This also means that what you or any author to whom you refer might *believe* is also out. Researchers need more than belief to go on.

Suggested reading

The following is not intended as a comprehensive reading program. It includes a number of books that we and our own students have found most useful, but it does not by any means cover the enormous range of literature on methodology and method that might be canvassed. We intend only to indicate a number of possible starting points, points from which you will in all likelihood diverge as you start to refine your own research design.

Research methodology (general)

Crotty, M. (1998) *The foundations of social research: Meaning and perspective in the research process* has the same sort of appeal as Blaikie and Flick. Crotty also has a good chapter on phenomenology if you are thinking of this as your methodology.

Flick, U. (2007) *Designing qualitative research* takes the same sort of approach in the *Introduction to Qualitative Research.*

Research methodology (specific)

You and your supervisors will discuss the methodology that you will use. One of the reasons that you have the supervisor(s) that you do is their expertise in relation to a particular methodology, and they will advise you on your reading on this aspect of preparation for your Confirmation of Candidature.

If you are taking up **poststructuralism**, you might be referred to the work of a number of authors:

1. If you are directed to Foucault:
   Foucault, M. (1973) *Discipline and punish: The birth of the prison.* Penguin: London.
   Perhaps something like McHoul and Grace's (1993) *A Foucault primer: Discourse, power and the subject* will help you to engage Foucauldian concepts at the outset of your studies.
2. You might also be referred to other key texts by scholars like Lyotard and Derrida:
   Lyotard, J.-F. (1984) *The postmodern condition: A report on knowledge.*
   Derrida, J. (1973) *Speech and phenomena.*
3. Feminist theory might take your reading to Weedon:
   Weedon, C. (1988) *Feminist practice and post-structuralist theory* (an excellent book on poststructuralist theory in its own right).
4. If you are taking up **phenomenology**, then you cannot go past van Manen as a starting point:
   van Manen, M. (1990) *Researching lived experience: Human science for an action-sensitive pedagogy.*

5. For **symbolic interactionism**, a good introduction is Charon:
   Charon, J. M. (2009) *Symbolic interactionism: An introduction, an interpretation, an integration.*

Research method

Cohen, Manion, and Harrison (2000): *Research methods in education* gives a number of research methods appropriate to the sort of research we do, as well as canvassing strategies appropriate to method.
Silverman's (2003) *Doing qualitative research: A practical handbook* is exactly what the title suggests...a practical handbook that cuts straight to the essence of each point that he raises.

There are many texts that give you excellent information and advice on research method, but at this stage of your candidature you are not required to go into great detail in discussion of the method you will use. Neither will you be required to go into great detail on validity. Such things will be carefully considered when you are designing your research and writing your thesis. A more detailed selection for recommended reading is given at "Milestone 5: Methodology" chapter.

As you write this document, you will become familiar with conventions of research writing that you will go on to apply to the writing of your thesis. They may appear to be a matter of minutiae to you at this stage, but they are important for the production of a professional piece of research writing acceptable to other members of the research community to which you are seeking entry.

Handling the minutiae

By the time you have competed your Confirmation of Candidature, you will have learned a great detail of the minutiae involved in research writing for examination. It is worth your while to reflect on some of these, as they are details that will make your thesis so much more appealing to an examiner. If your supervisor is a good editor, this will have been picked up on in various drafts of your document. If not, some things might have got past at this stage, but they will not in the thesis. Examiners are most particular about what is acceptable in a thesis. Below are some of those details that we have constantly dealt with in our students' work.

Conventions of writing

1. There is only one space between a full stop and the first word of the next sentence, not two. It used to be two spaces when people used typewriters, but word processors take care of the size of spaces.
2. There is to be no use of contractions or abbreviations in formal writing. You do not use contractions such as *don't, couldn't, won't, shouldn't've*. You will write them all in full: *do not, could not, will not, should not have*. You will not use *ie, eg, etc*. You will write these in full as well: *that is, for example,* and if you must, *etcetera*, but better to write *and so on*. (We have had a candidate required to change every single contraction and abbreviation in the thesis because the examiner said so.)

3. If you don't know the correct use of the apostrophe look it up before you insert one ... don't guess. Better still, so that you don't have to look it up each time, learn the rules for its use. It is not hard.
4. When it comes to punctuation, you can get by with commas and full stops only. It is easier to write interesting sentences if you can also use em-dashes, colons, and semicolons, but if you do not know the rules and conventions for their use, do not use them. We find constantly that our students are putting them into their work in complete ignorance of how to use them. If you do not know, find out. Again, it is not hard.

Inappropriate expressions

There are words that you will use in everyday conversation and not think twice about doing so. You cannot do this with the same abandon when writing your thesis, for example:

- *this correlates with*: Cannot be used because it is an expression that has specific meaning in using statistics, and in your qualitative research, it does not apply. Use *this is consistent with...*
- *this aligns with*: More awkward than incorrect. Again, use *this is consistent with...*
- *it is a problematic* (whatever): Usually, this word is used incorrectly to say that something is a *problem*. The problematic has a specific meaning in research writing. When researchers problematize something, they take an everyday situation or event and apply theory to it as part of analyzing it. Lack of parking may be problem. Lack of parking is problematic when we frame it as deliberate government policy to discourage the use of private cars and construct it as a social experiment.
- *recent studies have shown*: Just too vague. First, you need to cite the research to which you are referring. Second, your thesis will be published some time hence, and the idea of what is recent may well have no relevance when it is. Not only that, but anyone reading your thesis years hence will have no idea when this *recent* is. An examiner would be disinclined to accept this. Give the year(s) of publication.
- *it seems/it appears that*: Also too vague for research writing. You would be expected to be more definite in what you say.
- *many, more, most, the majority, often, very*...all such words are just too vague to be used in serious research writing, so drop them from your PhD vocabulary.
- *it is important/vital/essential*: Just think what these words mean. Then don't use them in research writing. How can you establish what *importance* is? If it is *vital*, it is necessary to life, and may do in medical research writing, but not in yours. *Essential* is just too vague to be used.
- *in terms of*: Watson (2005) gives this phrase as one of his examples of weasel words, ones that serious writers ought to avoid. Try *in relation to* instead. And if you have time, we recommend that you consult this book as it is full of good advice to the writer of a thesis.

Word use

Know the meanings and correct use of the words that you select:

- *utilize* and *usage* do not mean the same as *use*. Incorrect use of *utilize* and *usage* can be easily avoided. Select the correct word, the one that you mean: *use*.

- *differing* does not mean the same as *different.* Incorrect use of *differing* can also be easily avoided. Use the correct word: *different.*
- there are rules for the use of *among* and *amongst.* Unless you know and apply these rules, you will usually be wrong when you use *amongst.* You will always be right if you use *among.* The same applies to *while* and *whilst,* so always use *while* if you don't know the rules. You can always learn them…it's not hard.
- *definitive*: You mean *definite,* so write *definite.*
- *practice* is a noun; *practise* is a verb

  advice is a noun; *advise* is a verb

  council is a noun; *counsel* is a verb

The use of the ***c*** and the ***s*** gives you an important clue here. Each word is spelt correctly, but each has a different meaning, and this is not difficult to learn either.

Paragraphing

One of the first things that you will have learned in writing your Confirmation of Candidature document is that in academic writing, one sentence is NOT a paragraph. It is in newspapers and magazines, and often in textbooks. A thesis is part of the academic writing genre and conventions of the genre apply. Attention paid to paragraphing means that you keep your writing on track, and that track is to address all that you write to your research questions.

A paragraph has at least four sentences, and each sentence in the paragraph has a particular function. There may be many more sentences, but the minimum number is four. The first sentence is the topic sentence. In your case, it is the topic of this chapter, this section, or this subsection in relation to your research question(s), so refer to it quite specifically in this sentence. The sentence, or more likely sentences, that follow this explain or develop aspects related to that topic sentence in some detail. The next sentence or sentences will refer to appropriate literature or data to support what you are claiming in this paragraph. You will NEVER write a paragraph that does not refer to the literature or your data in some part of it. The last sentence will refer to the topic sentence again and provide a link to the next paragraph, making a neat parcel of writing that maintains its relevance and keeps both you and the reader (your examiner(s) in this case), on track. The structure is inherent to the genre of academic writing.

Consider the fairy tale for a moment. The genre is a well-established one, with accepted and expected features of structure, style, and language. The opening sentence (the equivalent of the topic sentence) always begins with *Once upon a time.* Subsequent details are always present: the poor person being helped in some way, a bit of magic, perhaps some talking animals, some forces of the wicked being overcome by some forces of the good. These are the equivalent of the explanation, development, and supporting the claims made sentences in your paragraphs. The final sentence is always *And they all lived happily ever after.* This is the equivalent of the final sentence of your academic paragraph. If you take up such an idea of the genre and apply it throughout your research writing, your path will be a smooth one as far as structuring your writing is concerned. One of our students has found this a helpful analogy in structuring her writing. She calls it *The Fairy Tale Principle*.

Signposting

Another thing that you will have learned is the importance of signposting for the examiner(s). Careful attention to paragraphing means that you are always reminding the examiner(s), and yourself, of the direction that your thesis is taking, keeping the research question(s) before them as they read and before you yourself as you write. Applying this same principle to an entire chapter, sections, and subsections means that the focus on the research questions is maintained. It means that relevance is maintained. Good thesis writing is explicit in its presentation of the research being written up. Unless you make it clear to the examiner(s), they will not know just how relevant what you are writing is, for none if it is self-evident as far as the reader is concerned.

You will use topic sentences to lead the reader into a particular aspect of your research, and you will use your final sentences to round things off for them and provide a link to what is yet to come. Your opening and ending sentences of the chapter will do the same thing. A good rule of thumb, too, is never to finish a section or subsection of a chapter without an explicit reference to your research questions.

Suggested reading

Zeegers (2013) *Grammar matters* deals with the basic grammar knowledge that you need to write correctly and with confidence.

Structuring the program of study

As you have successfully completed your Confirmation of Candidature, you are at the point where you start to extend and deepen your understanding of the literature on research, as well as the literature on research that has been or is being conducted in the field you are investigating. That sort of understanding will help you in writing the application for ethics clearance for what you are proposing to do. Generally, your ethics application will be your next milestone reached. You will not be doing this in isolation from other activities engaged in doing your PhD, for what you read on methodology will inform your considerations of method, which will inform what you decide regarding technique, all of which will inform what you put into your ethics application.

Given this, it is appropriate to note that the milestones considered in the following sections are not to be seen as sequential steps toward achieving your PhD goal. There will be considerable overlap as you tackle each one over the next two or three years. While each is singled out for separate discussion, in the undertaking of each you will double up on some, focus on one for a while before going back to reconsider another, and so on. You will compose your ethics application, for example, but still be doing reading on technique, or method, or methodology at the same time. Even so, it would be worth your while to set out the structure of your thesis so that you may structure your program of reading and writing accordingly. A suggested structure is given below, but we would stress that this is not in any way prescriptive. You may set your thesis out in any way that you like, but it will probably look something like this:

Chapter 1 Situating the Study (see "Milestone 11: Finishing, submitting and examination" chapter for detail on writing this chapter)
Chapter 2 Literature Review
Chapter 3 Methodology
Chapter 4 Method (You would include discussions of ethics and validity in this chapter)
Chapter 5 Data Gathering
Chapter 6 Data Analysis
Chapter 7 Recommendations and Conclusions

The milestones which follow in this book reflect this sort of structure, but we all structure our programs differently. It is unlikely that you will proceed on a step by step basis. It is likely that you will be doing several things at the same time. You may work on the literature review over the whole course of the study, keeping it relevant and up to date, and make an ethics application and start generating data early on. You may find it advisable, though, to have your methodology chapter well advanced before you start your interviews, surveys, questionnaires, or whatever data-gathering technique you will use (which is what we would recommend). You will in all probability take breaks from various elements to keep your mind fresh by focusing on something else for a while. The point to be made is that each of these milestones is to be reached at some point, and when each has been reached, it will all come together and you will have a thesis to be bound and submitted for examination within the next two or three years.

Conclusion

Your Confirmation of Candidature is a major milestone reached. Depending on the terminology used at your university, it takes you from a Provisional Candidate (or an equivalent concept) to a Confirmed Candidate (or equivalent concept), on your way toward getting your PhD. In reaching this milestone, you have learned a good deal about what it means to complete your PhD. Taking this on board, you will proceed toward your next milestones relatively unfettered by what may be time-consuming attention to details of incorrectness and noncompliance with conventions of research writing. It will save a good deal of time as you will not have to do so much editing and correcting. You have been through a preliminary examination on your research, determining your written and oral skills in relation to getting your PhD, and you have not been found wanting. This should provide a real fillip to your undertaking. Now the real work begins.

Hot Tip 2

Start your PhD bibliography using the bibliographic software made available to you through the university. Your university will provide licenses for software that you may download at no cost to you, such as *EndNote* or *RefWorks*. If you are not sure how to use them, get to the workshops on bibliographic software provided by the university right away. Do not put this off for a moment. Then be really disciplined and spend some time each week entering your references. If your university does not provide such access, apply for funds from your Research and Graduate Office or Graduate School administration to purchase the software, as it is essential to your being able to generate a correctly formatted bibliography or references list in accordance with the Style specified by your university. If neither of these options is available to you, we strongly recommend that you purchase it in some other way, for you really do need this for your PhD. Do not imagine that you will be able to deal with your references manually…you are guaranteed to get them wrong if you try this, and it may take you weeks or even months that would be better spent on the body of the Confirmation of Candidature document, and later the thesis.

Milestone 3: Getting ethics clearance

3

Why ethics?

Given that you are a qualitative researcher within an interpretivist tradition who is investigating a social world, you will be working with people participating in your research. This means that you need ethics clearance before you proceed with any generation of data in relation to these participants. You do not need ethics clearance for working with public documents that are readily accessible, but you do if you are intending to access people's files, letters, diaries, journals, and so on that are not in the public domain. The design of your research has already taken this into account (see "Milestone 2: The confirmation or defence of candidature" chapter), and now that you have reached this chapter, you will give issues of ethics more detailed consideration.

What ethics clearance is

In all of our dealings in life, we try to behave ethically. This means that our behavior toward others is unimpeachable: we are moral; we are honest; we do not put others in harm's way, physically, emotionally, or psychologically. We are able to be trusted, in fact. Most of the time, this is implicit in all that we do. When it comes to conducting research, though, it is explicit. It ought to go without saying that your research must not breach any laws, but human behavior does encompass more than that which is lawful, and this is where ethics comes in. We make it clear to others in our research community and in our community of research participants that the research that we are undertaking is moral, honest, not putting anybody in harm's way, physically, emotionally, or psychologically. We will, in fact, do no harm. These three words of doing no harm encapsulate the reasons for having our research cleared by others involved in the research field. In order to have our research acceptable to and accepted by the wider research community, we are required to have what we are doing scrutinized and assessed as being in accordance with research ethics principles and protocols.

The ethics committee

We are given ethics clearance by a committee of people who apply specific and explicit ethics principles in their reading of what it is that we propose to do. This committee will usually include members of the public not necessarily involved in active research in any way. The person on the top of the Clapham bus comes to mind here;

that person is simply a reasonable member of the community. It will usually include active researchers, even if not necessarily in your field of research. It may or may not include other PhD candidates as student representatives. Some may be elected representatives from the academic staff of the university. Others may have been nominated from outside the university. The point of this is that the research is to be seen in the light of what constitutes ethics in relation to your selection of paradigm, methodology, method, technique, and so on. You may have particularly clever things in mind for gathering and analyzing your data, but that is not the ethics committee's concern. Its concern is entirely that your selections in relation to what you are proposing conform with the requirements of explicit ethics requirements, in accordance with published official policy and statements regarding ethics in your country.

These are so important that they are formulated and articulated at government levels. Some form of a Human Research Ethics Committee (HREC) will have been put in place by your university, and it will have established procedures first of all for its own operations, membership, application forms, meetings and meeting their conduct requirements, and so on. These will have been based on the country's policy and policy statements on ethics in the conduct of research. It may be of some interest to you as a researcher to be part of the whole thing. If you find that your university's ethics committee is looking for student representatives, you might seek nomination for election by your peers. You may also do this if you are already an academic staff member undertaking a PhD.

Ethics clearance and your research

Governments, universities, and researchers themselves take ethics most seriously, as will you. Getting ethics clearance is not just a hurdle to jump before you proceed; it is a very real commitment to that notion of doing no harm. You submit what you propose to a number of others with a similar commitment to the notion that your proposed research behavior may be examined from the number of perspectives that they offer. You will have consulted your supervisor(s) on the research design and they will have offered insights on ethics considerations, and now you will have the insights of others as well. Some universities require that all who submit applications undertake some form of training or a short course on ethics and research, with an official pass result before they will even accept an application. You need to allow for this when you devise your research schedule. The end result will mean that you may proceed with confidence that your research indeed does meet the required standards of ethics. Then you write your application.

Identify potential problem areas

The *do no harm* expression is a good guide in preparing your application, but it is possible that you have not taken into account all that this may involve. It is far better to identify potential problem areas before submitting an application to an ethics committee. The following deals with interview possibilities only, but may also apply to other means of data collection, such as surveys, or written responses to questions, or responses to material read, displayed, or recited to people.

You may want to interview or survey perpetrators of violence, but in asking them about their perpetrations you may be asking them to incriminate themselves as law-breakers, especially if you are referring to violence they have perpetrated but have apparently got away with so far.

You may want to interview or survey victims of crime, but in doing so you may be subjecting them to unpleasant memories of what had happened to them and so cause emotional distress.

You may want to interview or survey minors without their parents' or caregivers' presence or consent, and in doing so be in breach of ethics principles yourself if the ethics committee has not given clearance to do this.

You may want to interview or survey members of a minority group within your society, and in doing so breach that minority's own social code (members who may not be allowed to speak on certain or taboo subjects, or women on their own, or people who may be particularly vulnerable in the wider community, and so on).

You may consider that interviewing or surveying your colleagues, for example, may not cause them to become ill or disadvantaged, but you need to consider whether or not they may become stressed because of some personal reaction to the subject of interview questions, or worse still, that there may be implied criticism of your or their employer that may do them harm when it comes to promotion, daily interactions between staff, and so on.

You may want to interview or survey your underlings, such as students or employees, thinking that they will do this quite freely as you are not forcing them to participate, but there is an implied coercion here in that they may feel that given your status, they will be somehow disadvantaged by you if they decline.

You may not even want to interview or survey any or all of these people, but want to ask them to provide you with contact details of others (their family, friends, other members of their communities, colleagues, clients, patients, and so on) by means of such things as access to office lists, data bases, rolls, and personal communications, which means that confidentiality agreements or privacy laws may be breached.

There are concerns about doing no harm in all such examples, but this does not mean that you cannot research in such areas with such people. What it means is that you are to anticipate that there may be problem areas and put things in place to deal with them. This is not say that you are dealing with an administrative hurdle, but that you demonstrate your own commitment to acting in accordance with ethics requirements not only in doing no harm, but indeed your respect for your research participants and their rights. That concern extends to the fact that people who volunteer to participate in your research may simply be inconvenienced in some way by making the time and effort to do what you are inviting them to do.

Writing the application for ethics clearance

In the case of the PhD candidate submitting an application to an ethics committee, the principal supervisor is the principal researcher, even though it is you conducting the actual research. The principal supervisor is responsible for what research is to be conducted, and so is responsible for it being conducted in compliance with ethics requirements. They will read what you write in the application, probably comment on it and ask for amendments so that they can sign it off before it goes to the ethics committee.

i. For the Ethics Committee Members

When you write the application, you will write it in the format and on the forms required by your ethics committee. You will follow the instructions to the letter, not leaving any sections blank, nor questioning why any particular items might be considered necessary by the ethics committee. Just tell the committee what you are going to do, how you are going to do it, how nobody will be harmed in any way, where you have identified potential problems, and how you propose to address them.

The committee will want to have a description of your research couched in what they would designate as lay terms. This is exactly what it means. The committee is made up of a number of people with different backgrounds; not all are active or even retired researchers themselves, and even if they are, they are not necessarily knowledgeable in your field. Many are wider community members with an interest in what we do; only some are academics or researchers themselves. Many are retired from professions such as nursing, teaching, the law, and the police force, and some are not professionals at all. Others may be temporarily out of the workforce. They are in the main lay people, so describe your research so that they can understand it. An example is given below:

> *The project will explore undergraduate students' responses to a teaching and learning strategy of group work as part of their studies. Students will be invited to evaluate their group work activities as individuals and groups. The evaluation will be on the basis of explicit directions regarding what is expected of members of a group undertaking studies in their subject areas. They will be separate groups of students in the Schools of Education, Behavioural Science and Social Sciences, Nursing, Psychology, Science, Physical Education, and Engineering. They will be drawn from First, Second and Third Years in these Schools.*

The ethics committee will want to know why you are conducting this research. A response like, "to get my PhD" does not help them in determining the ethics implications of what you are doing, so again, be clear about this. Tell them, in lay terms, the aims, research objectives key research questions, and significance of the project you want to undertake:

> *This research seeks to gain a deeper understanding of the requirements for more effective integration of group work in teaching and learning for students who will enter the professions when they graduate, an approach which a review of the literature suggests is innovative within modes of university education (see for example [citation]). It will investigate the strategy of teaching effective group work behaviour to students. A review of the literature on group work has shown that both students and their lecturers and tutors consistently state their aversion and even outright resentment of group work (citation). The literature has also highlighted the need for further research in this area. This research is being undertaken at the same time that professional organisations and course accreditation bodies require that group work be included at least as a part of the study that their future professionals undertake (citation from the relevant professional/accreditation organisations here). This project will explore the possibilities of explicit teaching of effective group work to students, who will then engage a group work study exercise. These students are in*

effect undergraduate professionals, and the research will determine the success or otherwise of such a teaching and learning strategy when it is applied to a group work exercise conducted for the purpose of this research.

This is all pretty straightforward. That person on the top of the Clapham bus will be able to see what is intended, but then they will want to know how you will get your data on this issue. Keeping them in mind as the audience for your writing, tell them:

The research will be based on data collected from student participants in number a of focus groups run by an independent and experienced focus group conductor who will also record the sessions for later transcription by the researchers. Student participants will be invited to give oral responses to the ways in which the tutor in each class has taught effective group work strategy, and ways in which they have been able to apply effective group work strategy in class. No student in any of the classes will be required to participate; all will be invited but only volunteers will form the focus groups. The researchers will analyse the transcripts of student responses, examining the language students use. In doing this, they will identify similarities and differences in student responses to their experience of group work.

It is possible that your ethics committee, with its focus on lay membership, will still see research as being setting a hypothesis to be proved, and ask for one. Many lay people and even academics consider that if there is no hypothesis to be tested there is no research happening, so just tell them that your type of research deals with research questions to be explored. They will also want to know what benefits will result from it. If you cannot identify benefits to flow from this research to the ethics committee, you will be unlikely to get ethics approval, for if there is no benefit for anyone from this research, it is not only a waste of time but also a lack of respect for the participants. This is not acceptable as far as ethics are concerned:

The research will be of benefit not only to the planning of teaching and learning at the University, but also to wider education. More particularly, it will be of benefit to professional education communities, given their concern with this aspect of undergraduate preparation for entry to their professions.

A major concern of ethics committees is the ways in which participants will be recruited. Are you, for example, looking to work with vulnerable or exploitable or underage or elderly or disabled people? Are you looking to work with socially marginalized or minority groups, such as members of your country's Indigenous communities, or travelers? Do you wish to approach convicted criminals or their victims? Make it clear who you will be inviting to participate and how you will get in touch with them. Make it clear also how you intend to ensure their anonymity. While statistics and associated issues of sample size in relation to an identifiable group is usually not a concern of ours, do not assume that the ethics committee will know this: tell them.

Tell them your proposed recruitment method, which is also a major concern of the committee. How will you get their contact details, such as their addresses, e-mail contacts, or phone numbers? Do you intend to access an organization's databases? If you do, how will you be able to get access to them in ways that conform with ethics requirements? Even if you work for the organization whose members you intend to investigate, and you have regular and endorsed access to the files as part of your normal duties, you can't assume that you can use the details in those files for the purposes of your research. That would be a breach of ethics. If we follow the examples given so far, we would say something like the following:

> *All students enrolled in the units concerned will be invited to participate in the research. Given this, they do not form a sample size but rather a representative group of students across a number of classes and units at the university engaged in a particular form of group work activities.*

Where you do want access to an organization's files, you will first of all secure the approval of the organization concerned and attach a copy of the letter to this effect to your application. You will organize this in such a way as to ensure that the participants retain their anonymity, and participate only in a voluntary capacity. To the committee, you will say something like:

> *[Name of the organisation] will invite their memberships to participate in a questionnaire as voluntary participants in the research. They will do this via their email list and newsletters. Participants will volunteer to complete the questionnaire by accessing the online link provided in the emails and newsletters.*

Another area of concern for an ethics committee is that of inducement to participate. You would be wise to avoid any suggestion whatsoever of financial or other inducements to participate, unless of course you have a deliberate strategy of inducement here (even if it is a chocolate frog, a dinner for focus groups members, book vouchers, cinema tickets, and so on). We all really would prefer to see volunteers, but it may be the case that you want to research the types of people that respond to inducements to participate in research, or indeed the inducements themselves as effective or not in having people decide to participate. Whatever the part that inducement plays, it is just a matter of stating exactly what it is, and how it is to be accessed by or given to participants. What is a more likely situation, though, is that you will arrange for costs incurred by participants, such as travel costs. You may also be giving equipment or tools to participants, for recording things, for example. Such things are to be noted and their role fully explained as being part of the research design and procedures to be used.

A step beyond the issue of inducement is that of coercion, always a matter of concern for researchers and ethics committees. You really do want to have voluntary participation so that your research is not clouded in any way. Your reading of the research literature will already have told you that all researcher and participant relationships are unequal. This is a given. The question then becomes one of whether you will you be using this to coerce participation, and of course the answer is, "No." Your ethics committee has a slightly different focus from that of the research literature, and will accept your "No," or your "No" with qualifications. You may be researching with your own student, client, patient or underling base, which clearly shows that the participants are dependent on you in some way. One way that you may deal with this is to indicate how the relationship is not affecting the research in any way. In the case of students, for example, you may design the research to be done once their time with you as their teacher is over. Another way may be to employ a professional facilitator or independent data gatherer while using pseudonyms and codings to ensure complete anonymity of the participants. This way, you will never know who participated and who did not.

Another thing that the ethics committee will want to know is what questions you are going to ask your participants. If you intend to interview, you will include a list of the interview questions, with the proviso that these are open-ended, and that you will allow for follow-up questions for elaboration or clarification of responses that you anticipate you will receive. If you are going to be using a survey or a questionnaire, you will attach a copy for the committee to peruse. You will not have any questions of the "When did you stop beating your wife?" type, because these are not up to ethics standards. You will not try to trick or trap any participant, and you will not interview in a surreptitious way, such as using hidden cameras or microphones, unless these are integral to your research and you can make a convincing, scholarly case for the ethics committee.

It is not only a matter of ethics, but also a matter of respect for participants, to make provision for their being informed of research results, usually in the form of work published out of the data that they have provided. You will probably write conference papers and journal articles along the way to submitting your thesis, but the main publication will be your thesis, and perhaps later the book that comes out of it. You will write something like:

> *It is anticipated that the results will be disseminated initially in the form of research conference presentations, after which they will form the basis of publications in international refereed journals. The main means of dissemination is in the form of a thesis produced by the student researcher. It is also possible that a book may result from the project.*

The ethics committee will then want to know what you are going to do to inform participants of just what they are in for if they take up your invitation. The word to stress here is *invitation*. You will not say that you will *ask* or *require* or *need* their participation. You will only say that you invite it. You will include a copy of the document, usually a letter or an e-mail message, inviting participation and explaining what you intend to do, why you intend to do it, and how you intend to do it. You will make it clear that this is purely voluntary, and that participants may withdraw at any time with no adverse consequences to themselves, up until the time that data are aggregated and individual responses will no longer be able to be identified. Once the pseudonyms, codings, and so on go into your planned aggregation for analysis, you will not know whose responses are whose and you will not be able to pull a particular response or set of responses out of that aggregation.

You will explain what they are invited to do, in what circumstances, conditions, or places, and how long it will take. You will advise them of counseling or support services available to them should they feel that they require it. The point to note here is that if they feel that they require it, that is all that matters. They decide this; you do not. You will advise them that the research is to be conducted in accordance with ethics committee approval, and within the limits of the law. This last point is of some significance, for if you come across instances of criminal activity, you are required by law to report it. You cannot be part of a cover up of child abuse, for example. You will provide contact details of the principal researcher and the ethics committee contact person. Having written your letter, you will attach it to your application.

Some organizations require separate ethics applications to conduct research with those for whom they are responsible. Education departments, for example, require that potential researchers make ethics applications directly to them, as well as to the university concerned. Where you want to access a group that has been identified in your own community as requiring particular attention in relation to research and the ethics consideration of it, you will show how you have addressed this requirement. Your first concern, of course, is that members of such a community will be treated as they ought, as specified. To illustrate this, we have used an Australian example that pertains to research with Indigenous Australian peoples, by the Australian Institute for Aboriginal and Strait Islander Studies (2012), given below. Other countries will have similar statements of principles and guidelines for researchers. These are to be consulted before submitting a proposal to the relevant ethics committee, and indeed, before conducting such research. There is a significant point in relation to the example used here: ethics clearance is to be sought from the Institute itself, and this will be in addition to the application to your university one. In some cases, you will be required to apply for ethics clearance for your proposed research *before* you submit one to your university. You will need to check such requirements and comply with them.

Australian Institute of Aboriginal and Torres Strait Islander Studies Principles of ethical research

Principle 1: Recognition of the diversity and uniqueness of peoples, as well as of individuals, is essential.
Principle 2: The rights of Indigenous peoples to self-determination must be recognized.
Principle 3: The rights of Indigenous peoples to their intangible heritage must be recognized.
Principle 4: Rights in the traditional knowledge and traditional cultural expressions of Indigenous peoples must be respected, protected, and maintained.
Principle 5: Indigenous knowledge, practices, and innovations must be respected, protected, and maintained.
Principle 6: Consultation, negotiation, and free, prior and informed consent are the foundations for research with or about Indigenous peoples.
Principle 7: Responsibility for consultation and negotiation is ongoing.
Principle 8: Consultation and negotiation should achieve mutual understanding about the proposed research.
Principle 9: Negotiation should result in a formal agreement for the conduct of a research project.
Principle 10: Indigenous people have the right to full participation appropriate to their skills and experiences in research projects and processes.
Principle 11: Indigenous people involved in research, or who may be affected by research, should benefit from, and not be disadvantaged by, the research project.
Principle 12: Research outcomes should include specific results that respond to the needs and interests of Indigenous people.
Principle 13: Plans should be agreed for managing use of, and access to, research results.
Principle 14: Research projects should include appropriate mechanisms and procedures for reporting on ethical aspects of the research and complying with these guidelines.

We have also included an example of one candidate's successful response to this set of principles when it was submitted to their ethics committee.

Annotated example 1

Clear indication that not all principles apply

Direct and explicit reference to the stipulated resource re ethics requirements for research on a particular community group

The principles stated by the Australian Institute of Aboriginal and Torres Strait Islander Studies Principles of Ethical Research that directly relate to this research project are listed below, as well as the risk management procedures that will be put in place to deal with the identified risks.

- Principle 3: The rights of Indigenous peoples to their intangible heritage must be recognised.

This principle will be addressed in the research project by the researchers proceeding on the understanding that Indigenous peoples have the right to maintain, control, protect and develop their cultural heritage, traditional knowledge and manifestation of their sciences. The researchers will not harass or seek any knowledge that may be considered sacred or not available to be disseminated to people outside the community.

- Principle 5: Indigenous knowledge, practices and innovations must be respected, protected and maintained.

This principle will be addressed in this research project by the researchers making clear to Aboriginal participants that once Aboriginal knowledge is recorded, it becomes property as defined under Western laws and concepts. As they do so, the researchers will recognise and protect the knowledge of Aboriginal peoples throughout the project.

Each principle not only listed but discussed re ways to address it

Principles relevant to this research identified and cited in their entirety

- Principle 6: Consultation, negotiation and free, prior and informed consent are the foundation for research with or about Indigenous peoples.

This principle will be addressed in a number of ways:
1) Opportunity provided to have a Local Aboriginal Education Consultant Group (LAECG) member present during interviews.
2) Opportunity provided to have a member of their family or community present during interviews.
3) Counselling services provided by their respective Aboriginal community cooperatives to be available for access by participants. The counselling services will be informed of the interviews taking place at the time. Participants will also be advised of the possibilities of contacting Lifeline [phone number given]
4) The XXXX Aboriginal Education Association XXX (XAEAXXX) will be contacted for approval to conduct the interviews and notified when the interviews will take place.

- Principle 11: Indigenous people involved in research, or who may be affected by research, should benefit from, and not be disadvantaged by, the research project.

The researchers acknowledge that the research should benefit Aboriginal people at the local level. In order to demonstrate this, the researchers will discuss openly and negotiate with the communities any potential benefits and development aimed directly at and for the community. The researchers will discuss with Aboriginal communities the best ways in which the information gained from the research could be used to benefit those communities.

- Principle 13: Plans should be agreed for managing use of, and access to, research results.

The researchers will acknowledge the contributions of Aboriginal peoples by providing ongoing access for Indigenous people to access the research results. Before interviewing, the ownership of research results, including institutional ownership of data, individual rights of researchers and Indigenous participants will be mutually agreed upon in writing.

Additional procedures acknowledge need to consider mitigation of possible risks to participants

A process that the researchers will follow in order to mitigate any risks to Aboriginal participants associated with this research is to invite another member of the community in which the participant lives to be present at the interview. In addition Aboriginal community participants will be offered further assistance through the XXXX Consultant Groups (as identified by the XXXX).

Explicit reference to appropriate support organisation for this group

Citations given in the style required by that university.

It is to be noted that not every principle listed by IATSIS is applicable in this research project and only those that are have been addressed.

Annotated example 1 as a model

All participants, regardless of their affiliations, are to be treated in such ways as to minimize any risk to them as a result of participating in your research. With a generally straightforward one such as the group work research, this risk idea, however unlikely there is to be any harm done, is still to be addressed. Something like the following is required:

> *As the research is concerned with material produced after participants have completed the group work tasks, we do not anticipate that any potential risks will arise from participating in the project. We do see, though, that the publication of the research results could be potentially harmful if the participants were to be identified in any way. To minimise the risk of this, all participants will be referred to using pseudonyms and code names, and their surnames will never be referred to in any publication of research results. Participants will be assured that anonymity and confidentiality of participants will be maintained at all times during the project and in any publications arising from it.*

In writing their application to conduct research with Indigenous Australians, which was cleared by the ethics committee, this candidate has identified areas where the research relates to the principles stated, and notes that not each one of them applies. Where they do, though, the candidate has given some thought to ways in which they will be complied with in the conduct of this research. The example given below illustrates a number of ethics issues discussed in relation to this Milestone.

Annotated example 2

The title shows not one but two possible problem areas in relation to ethics. Can you identify them?

Title: Public and personal discourses: How 'teenage mothers' construct their parenting practices with their preschoolers

1. Teenagers include minors (under 18 or 21 years. 2. Mothers (minors) to address issues of very young children

Description: This research seeks to draw out the individual narratives of teenage mothers with a specific focus on their understandings of their literacy practices with their preschoolers in their home environment. A group of up to six participants will be invited to capture their own visual data of artefacts, events or actions that they perceive are linked to early literacy practices. The participants will be asked to take 40 to 50 photos and segments of video over a four to six week period. The participant-generated visual data will be used to elicit in-depth responses during two, one hour participant-centred, individual open-ended interviews with the researcher..

Claims made supported by citations

Non-specialist language for explanation

Aims: The aim of this research is to explore how teenage mothers construct their parenting practices to support the emerging literacy development in their preschooler's home environment. Parents play an important role in their children's emerging literacy development (*citations*). Early literacy development in preschoolers has been linked to cognitive and academic success in later years of schooling (*citation*). Entry to preschool and formal school settings can be problematic for some young children as they arrive with a diverse range of emerging literacy experiences. Some experiences are more highly valued within the dominant discourses of educators, and young children are "expected to exhibit many requisite skills prior to kindergarten" (*citation*). Such discourses may also be perpetuated in a range of ways, but may not represent the wide-ranging emerging literacy experiences facilitated in a diverse range of home environments. Some studies (*citations*) explore home literacy environments by asking parents to complete questionnaires or surveys focusing on the number of times they engage in specific literacy activities. However, the actual practices of the parents may not have been represented in the studies...

Clear statement of aims

Clear statement of what will be done

Significance: The study is significant as it will address gaps in the literature between the self-representation of teenage mothers and the policies, media and education discourses that position teenage mothers in particular ways. Much of the literature focuses on teenage mothers as a social problem and public discourses, in many instances, perpetuate particular negative constructions of teenage mothers (citations). Only a small number of studies have acknowledged the positive aspects of teenage motherhood and parenting practices and have used open-ended interviews to explore teenage mothers' perceptions and understandings of their localised contexts (citations).

Notes gaps in the literature re significance

Statement of benefit

It is anticipated that the knowledge generated from this research will offer new insights into teenage mothers' understandings of their parenting practices in relation to the emerging literacy development of their children. These insights will benefit the community by better informing policymakers and education decision makers at a national level…, as well as other groups in the wider community who work with or develop support programs for teenage mothers and their children.

Conduct of the research: The proposed methodology for this research is photo-elicitation. In photo-elicitation, visual data is used

Details procedures and processes

to guide the participant centred, individual open-ended interviews to elicit more in-depth responses. This technique assists the participants to direct the discussion and may encourage deeper conversations (*citations*). Photo-elicitation allows collaboration between the researcher and the participant, generating data that reflects the "participants' values, beliefs, attitudes, and meanings" (*citation*).

Data will be collected by participant-generated photography and video over a four to six week period. The data will be used to elicit in-depth responses in two, one hour, participant centred individual open-ended interviews.(*Citation*) suggests "the incorporation of self-made images by participants also creates an opportunity for the researcher to enter into participants' private worlds". Personal narratives generated from the data can more closely reflect the young women's world and the participants' personal voices can contribute to the research findings (*citation*). Open-ended interview questions provide broad parameters where the participants can formulate responses (*citation*). Participant centred open-ended interviews encourage dynamic interaction between the participant and the researcher (*citation*), thereby capturing the participant's perception, knowledge and experience.

Use of and reason for use of open ended questions

During an initial meeting, each participant will be given a digital camera, accessories, and an information sheet about how to collect the photos and video. The participants will be asked to take a series of 40 to 50 photos and segments of video of any artefact, event or action that they consider represents early literacy experiences with their preschoolers. The participants will have access to the camera and accessories for a period of four to six weeks to gather the visual data. At the end of the data gathering period, the researcher will collect the camera to download and copy the photos and video data. Pseudonyms will be allocated to each data set and the data coded. Each participant will receive a copy of their own self-generated data.

Anonymity of participants

The participant-generated photos and video will be the stimulus for the first, one hour participant-centred, individual open-ended interview. The interview will be recorded on a digital recorder and transcribed. Once the transcripts are prepared, each participant will receive a copy of their own transcript to read, and the researcher will return to conduct a second, one hour participant centred individual open-ended interview where participants will be invited to comment on the accuracy of the transcribed data and clarify responses from the first interview. This interview will also be recorded and transcribed. The participant-generated photos and video will also be available to support the participant's responses in the second interview. The photos and videos will not constitute research data, only the interview transcripts will be analysed.

Clear statement on how participants will be recruited

Recruitment: The researcher will seek out participants by advertising through a Young Parents Program in a regional city in XXX. The researcher has had initial informal contact with a program in the past and will make contact with the relevant parties to seek their permission to access the program to recruit participants to be part of the research. Up to six participants, aged between 15 and 19, will be invited to participate in this study. The specific age range has been chosen for this study as the young women who attend the Young Parents Program are in this age bracket. As this is a qualitative research project, a statistically representative sample

Position of researcher re recruitment

of the population is not required. Instead, the small sample of participants focuses on a specific local context to gain in-depth understandings and meanings of the participant's world (*citation*).

Includes benefits to participants themselves

Benefits of the research: It is anticipated that the knowledge generated from this research will offer new insights to teenage mothers' understandings of their parenting practices in relation to the emerging literacy development of their children. This is important as the children move towards more formal education contexts. These insights will benefit the community by better informing policymakers and education decision makers at a national level ..., as well as other groups in the wider community who work with or develop support programs for teenage mothers and their children.

States possible risks before addressing them

Risk management: This study has ethical considerations for the infants and preschoolers in the study as well as the teenage mothers. Although the young children could appear in the images taken by their mothers, there is no perceived harm to the young children as this is no different to having their photo taken or a video recorded in other situations. The participants who have volunteered to be part of the research process will themselves be contributing through the participant-generated photos and video that will be the stimulus for the participant centred, individual open-ended interviews. The perceived risk to the participants is through taking the time to take the photos and record the video, and being part of the interview process. According to the National Statement on Ethical Conduct in Human Research (2007) this could be categorised as inconvenience.

Refers to relevant document on ethics to support claims made

The participant generated data (photos and video) and audio taping of the interviews poses a potential risk to participants in terms of confidentiality. This risk will be managed by confidentiality procedures including the use of pseudonyms for participants and their children and the coding of the photographs and video segments. The participant-generated photos, video and all identifying information, transcripts and interpretations will be kept in separate locked facilities at the XXXX for a period of five years and will only be accessible to the Principal Researcher, Associate Researcher and student researcher. Participants will be informed of the security of the data through the and during the initial discussion. The participants can opt out of the research process at any time prior to the aggregation of data. The PLIS will provide a statement that indicates privacy and confidentiality is maintained under the legalities of law.

Plain Language Information Statement used

Details of procedures to reduce risk to participants

Photos and video will not be reproduced for publication at any time during the study or at the end of the study. The data are only used to elicit more in-depth responses for the participant centred, individual open-ended interviews which will be the basis for the analysis provided in the thesis. An information sheet will be given to each participant at an initial meeting detailing, that for confidentiality reasons, only photos of their own children are to be taken and to avoid all other people in the images.

Support to participants: It is not envisaged that additional support is necessary for participants as the collection of data through photography and video is not deemed to be harmful or cause risk to the participants as the type of task is within the context of normal activities the participants would engage in with their children.

> During the participant centred, individual open-ended interviews, teenage mothers will be asked to describe their parenting practices. This may generate feelings of anxiety because the participant may feel that comments she makes may be viewed negatively by the researcher. Where concerns may arise during the interviews, the researcher will immediately stop the interview. The participants will be given full details for contacting the Principal Supervisor if they have questions regarding the research or wish to discuss aspects of the research process. The 'Lifeline' phone number (XXXXXX) will be stated in the PLIS if participants feel they need to talk to a person who is trained to deal with issues that may affect them.

In spite of unlikelihood of their need, support mechanisms noted

Financial issues dealt with

> **Inducements/financial details**: Where required, travel costs will be reimbursed. Travel costs may occur for bus travel within the regional city. The researcher would envisage that this would be no more than $15 per participant distributed via a [*public transport electronic fare card*] and this will be determined once the participants consent to being part of the research.

References are also given in that University's References Style requirement.

The annotated examples as models

Both annotated examples were successful applications, receiving ethics clearance and enabling the candidates to proceed with their PhDs. An important point to consider in relation to any potential problems is that you say what they might be, however unlikely their eventuating, and what you have in place to deal with them. You may, even in relation to what seems the most innocuous of strategies, suggest the normally free counseling services offered by your university or the organization associated with the participants concerned. If there is an organization such as Lifeline available, you may refer to this as accessible by participants. In any case, ensure that you have given consideration to some sort of support for any participants that may for whatever reason imaginable become distressed or in some way discomfited by their participation. A reading of the ways in which the candidates in the annotated examples have set out their applications indicates that they have read the relevant policy documents and guidelines, have given careful consideration to issues of risk and risk management, and have been punctilious in addressing concerns that an ethics committee might have. They have shown themselves capable of managing ethics requirements for their proposed research. An added dimension to this, though, is the fact that they have named the principal researcher as the person ultimately responsible for the conduct of the research in relation to ethics considerations (as always required by ethics committees), and stated that they will receive constant monitoring from that supervisor as the research proceeds.

ii. For the Participants

(a) The Plain Language Information Statement, or the PLIS (or equivalent at your university) sets out what you have already set out for the ethics committee in even plainer language than you have already used for them. The idea is to ensure that participants are fully informed of what they are letting themselves in for. After the initial address to the participant, and the names of the researchers, you will give details of what will be done with the data, how it will be stored, when it will be destroyed, and so on. The following is a part of such a letter, which addresses what the relevant ethics committee has asked for:

> We are working together to find out XXX. We would like to invite you to participate in this project, where you would to allow us to record you and your child or the child in your care using the language that they normally use with you at home. We want to set these conversations around several types of talk that we think they might cover in their daily lives: Home Talk, Social Talk, School Talk, Teacher Talk. These conversations will be transcribed, and translated where necessary, and will give us data for a case study of such language use in our region. This research is important because, through the publication of results, it can contribute to improved practice in primary school literacy and language education as people come to understand more about language use. It is expected that each of you will spend about 45 minutes at the most talking to the researcher, with a number of precautions being taken to protect your identity and privacy and that of the child concerned.
>
> Each tape will be played back to you and the child so that you both know what is being used in the research, and if either of you does not want any part of it to be used, for any reason whatever (and these reasons do not have to be given), it will be left out. You will also be given a copy of the transcript of the taped conversations, and if you or your child do not want any of the material in the transcripts used, it will be struck off the transcript and not used. All of the information in transcripts or in publications will be presented in a way the does not reveal anyone's identity.
>
> All the information will be securely stored by the researcher in a locked filing cabinet in a locked office. Confidentially is assured, within the limits of the law. Tapes will be destroyed and transcripts shredded within five years of finishing this research. You are in no way obliged to take part, or to have your child or the child in your care take part in this research, and both you and they are free to withdraw any time during the research with no bad results to you.
>
> A copy of the research paper will be given to you at the end of the project so that you can view the results of the research.

You really do need to include this sort of statement

(b) Informed Consent

Now you are going to have to indicate to the ethics committee how you are going to establish that consent has formally and officially been given by an informed participant. Your letter will be accompanied by some means of indicating informed participant consent. Now, this may be on the basis of having returned a completed questionnaire or survey, or having accessed and completed an electronic survey instrument, or having signed a consent form. An informed consent form has a similar function to that letter that you are going to send, but it is a much briefer document. The form and format required will vary from one university to the next, but the example given below illustrates the point:

PROJECT TITLE: Give the same title as you have been using *throughout*

RESEARCHERS: *Give principal, associate and student researcher names*

Consent – Please complete the following information:

I, ... of ....

....

....

hereby consent to *(your name as student researcher and statement of what it is that you will be doing)*

The research project has been explained fully to me, verbally and/or in writing, and any matters on which I have sought information have been answered to my satisfaction.

I understand that:

Here is that type of statement again →

- all information provided by the participants will be treated with the strictest confidence (within the limits of the law) and data will be stored separately from any listing that includes their name and address
- participation in this research is voluntary
- aggregated results will be used for research purposes and may be reported in academic journals and texts, and at conferences
- there will be a recorded individual interview of approximately one hour's duration conducted
- the participants are free to withdraw their consent at any time during the study, in which event, their participation in the research study will immediately cease and any information obtained from it will not be used
- once information has been processed it is not possible to withdraw consent to participate.

SIGNATURE: .... DATE: ....

....

The words used

This application is quite separate from your thesis document. It is directed to a different audience for difference purposes from those of your thesis. First, you will write in future tense. Second, you will write in third person because you will be referring to a number of people involved in the research that you propose: the principal researcher; associated researcher(s); your associate supervisor(s); you, the student researcher; and the participants. You will say things like, "The student/the principal researcher will…"; "The participants will be invited to…" Other examples of words used are given below.

> *Risk management*: It is not anticipated that participants will face risks other than those associated with their normal daily professional activities, but any such risks that may emerge will be outweighed by the benefit to… (*and state what the benefits are*).

Support services for participants: While the researchers do not anticipate that there will be any need for additional support for participants, (*name the organization*) provides counseling services for its members, and all participants will be advised of the availability of these in the normal course of their time with this organization. Should participants indicate that they have a need for such support, they will be directed to those services. The researchers will also advise counselors that the project will be occurring at the times specified to alert them to any possible approaches that may be made by participants in relation to this project. Participants will be advised that should they suffer any discomfort or distress and feel they require additional support as a result of participation in this research, they will be referred to the free counseling services provided by the (*name the organization*) in their region or Lifeline on XXXX.

Informing participants of research outcomes, publications, and so on: All participants will be advised of the availability of any research publications that emerge from the project via a Web page launched for this purpose (*if this sort of thing is to be done).* Where copyright permits, copies of publications, seminar papers, and so on will also be posted on that Web page, available to any participants who wish to read them. The researchers anticipate that participants will be interested in what comes from the research, and will encourage all participants to maintain their interest in the project once it is finished.

Approval withheld

Not all applications receive clearance. If they are a blatant breach of established ethics requirements, they will not be cleared. This would suggest that the candidate has not given careful consideration of the ethics involved in conducting the research proposed. Not all are rejected out of hand, either. What usually happens is that the candidate has not been clear enough on aspects of detail, or has perhaps used language that might be suggestive of coercion (*asked/required to* rather than *invited*, for example), or has underestimated the possibilities of harm to participants invited to comment on their superiors, or has not timed the research to occur after a dependent relationship has ceased, or has even proposed asking participants with no known criminal record if they have ever committed a felony or a crime. In this last example, had the candidate been working with convicted criminals, they would have been able to make a case for putting such a question. This was not the case here. The candidate simply wanted to know if the participants' own experiences had influenced their current responses to the crime the researcher was investigating, and had felt that it was an innocent and legitimate question to ask. They had not read the policy statements regarding ethics in research carefully enough.

It is rare that an ethics committee will withhold clearance outright where the candidate has indicated that they have the sort of understanding of ethics requirements that the committee is looking for. While they would not clear a set of interview or survey questions regarding felonious or criminal behavior that was not shown to be integral to the research proposed, they will generally point to inappropriateness in terms used or incomplete detail regarding procedures to be engaged, and ask for clarification. This sort of thing will be addressed by the candidate, who will resubmit the application, or the questioned part(s) of the application, to reassure the committee members about their ethics concerns. The ethics committee will normally clear the proposed research at this point.

Suggested reading

The most important things for you to read in relation to your ethics application are the policy statements of your national government and your university in relation to ethics requirements, for your application will be written in accordance with stipulations provided in each of these.

Hot Tip 3

A former candidate, now a graduate, found themselves in the position of being able to, and wanting to, write a book out of the research undertaken during their PhD studies. When they checked their ethics application of the time, they found to their great relief that they had specified *book* as part of the publications of research results options. There had been no thought of a book in their mind at that time; they were only focussed on getting their PhD. Had they not specified the book option, they would not have been able to use the material from their PhD for the book. That person is now a published book author.

The ethics application form will ask you to specify the ways in which the research that you will conduct will be published. At this stage, you will probably feel comfortable specifying conference proceedings and journal articles along with the thesis itself. Remember the example of the candidate given above; specify the book as well, even if right now you have no intention of writing one. You will probably find that after having generated such a large amount of material that a PhD implies, and working through it as you analyze and discuss it, that you really do have more to say, and that a book would be the way to go about doing this. If you have ethics clearance for a book in which you use the data that you are about to collect, you don't have to do it all again when it comes to a book. And remember, you don't have to write a book. If you decide not to write one in the future, that's well and good. If you do decide to write one in the future, you have ethics clearance in place to do so.

Conclusion

Just as your Confirmation of Candidature is not to be seen as a hurdle, but as a chance to have knowledgeable scholars give careful consideration to your proposed research, so is your ethics application to be seen as an opportunity for you to have knowledgeable ethics committee members give careful scrutiny to your proposed research to ensure that it meets the required standards for what you propose to undertake. It is not to be seen as a hurdle to be cleared, but as a serious consideration for ensuring the highest standards of your work.

Part Two

Getting the PhD done

In "Milestone 2: The confirmation or defence of candidature" chapter, we looked at a diagram to help conceptualize the processes of the Confirmation of Candidature. We can now reconfigure it to help conceptualize the processes of the PhD itself.

The following milestones deal with each of these.

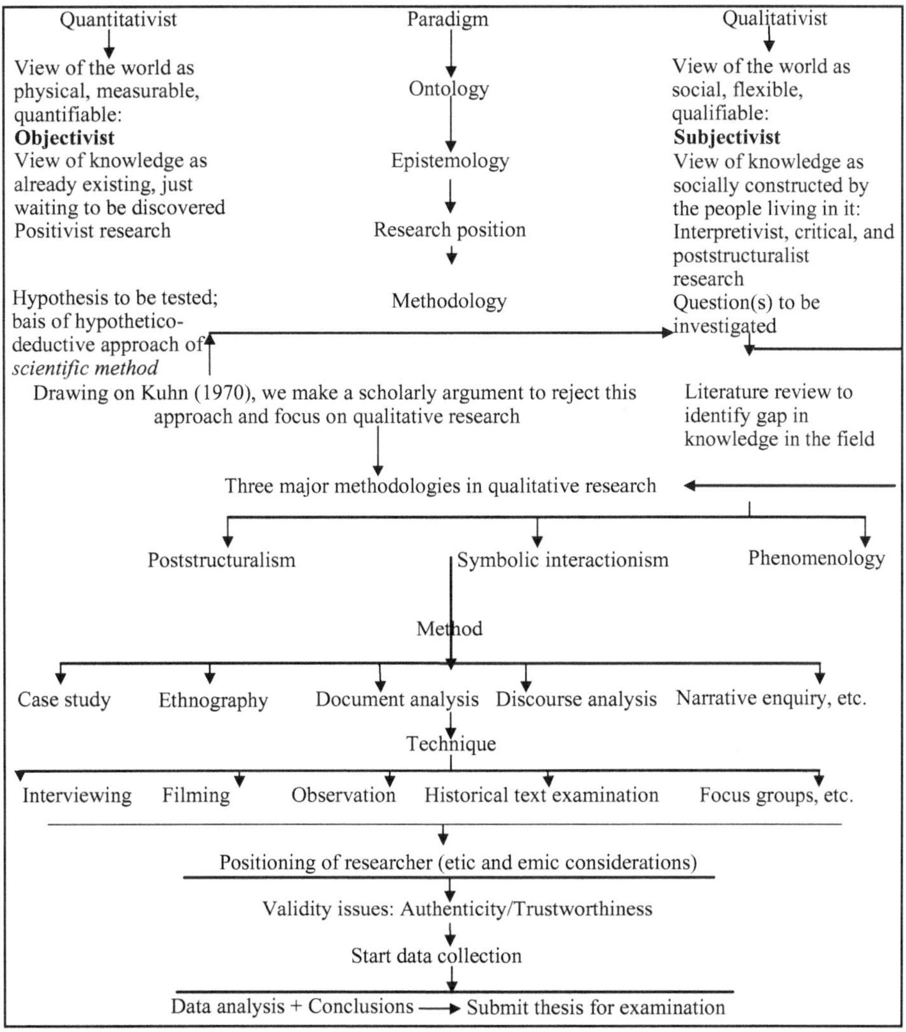

Milestone 4: The literature review

4

The literature review and your research

Here, we present just one of many possible strategies that a PhD candidate may use to prepare and write their literature review. Your candidature as a research student was endorsed because nobody else in the whole world who ever got to publish anything about this aspect of your field has looked at your chosen research question or issue from the perspective that you have. But your research is part of a bigger picture too, one that has developed a whole culture around research. Cooper (1989) makes the point, “Given the cumulative nature of science, trustworthy accounts of past research forms a necessary condition for orderly knowledge building” (p. 11). You will note that word *trustworthy* again. Your literature review is one of those trustworthy accounts of previous research. It is important to make this distinction between this literature being reviewed and other literature engaged in the course of the candidature. The literature on methodology and method, for example, will be used in the chapters that discuss these things. It will not be referred to in the writing of the literature review chapter. This chapter will deal specifically with the research that has already been done and published in the field being researched.

A problem area

Bruce (1994) argues that the research that she has done with research students at her university “suggests that supervisors of postgraduates and other teachers interested in the review process need to accept literature reviews as a problem area for students and develop strategies to help them” (p. 217). This would also suggest a need for you to talk to your supervisor(s) about any misgivings that you may have about attempting your literature review. Once a problem is identified, it can be managed. Most researchers are in the same position as you in starting a literature review from scratch, and in your case especially advice on where to start is not only most welcome but needed. The first thing that you need to establish is what the literature review is for, and what it does.

Bruce's research led her to identify six student conceptualizations of the literature review: as a list; as a search; as a survey; as a vehicle for learning; as a research facilitator; as a report. This indicates quite a range of conceptualisations in the students' minds, and what you think of the literature review at this stage of your candidature probably fits with one of these. She went on to classify these according to higher and lower level conceptualizations, arguing that the lower levels, perhaps understandable and predictable at the PhD candidate's early stages of study, are inadequate for the

Milestone Moments in Getting your PhD in Qualitative Research

Lower levels					Higher levels
List	**Search**	**Survey**	**Vehicle for learning**	**Research facilitator**	**Report**
No direct interaction between student and the literature	Lacking direct interaction: focus on the search process	More direct interaction: but unidirectional: focus on the literature itself	Direct interaction: focus beyond the literature and on student's own personal development	Direct interaction: added dimension of the impact of the literature on the research project	Direct interaction, but "terminal": ceases with the report; ceases to shape research and/or expand student's horizons

Figure 1 PhD candidate conceptualizations of the literature review.
Adapted from Bruce (1994).

full and rich engagement required at later stages. A diagrammatic representation of Bruce's suggested conceptualizations is shown in Figure 1.

You know better than anyone just where your understanding of the literature review fits in such a representation, and whether you need to adjust your own conceptualizations to higher levels or not. Circle the spot on the scale that best represents what you conceive of what the literature review is, then ask yourself how much more you need to find out.

What a literature review is

If you are operating at what Bruce considers the lower levels, you are probably about to launch into your 17,000-word chapter on all that you have read. If so, it is advisable that you reconsider just what it is that you are about to do. Your aim is to work at the higher levels on the scale. A literature review is by no means an exercise in cataloguing your reading over the past few weeks, or months, or years even.

A literature review presents an overview of issues in the field and their interrelationships. It identifies main concerns, findings, and common themes, but it also presents current debate on these. In doing so, it identifies limitations to the existing literature, and that is where you come in. You are not beginning a whole new area that nobody has ever considered before; you are examining one part of the field. You are not working on a Ground Zero basis; your research in your part of the field is what is new. What you find out is what will be part of a body of knowledge that others have generated up to this point.

Your contribution fits into this body of knowledge, but unless you explain this, nobody will know just how it does. When you write your literature review, take some pains to explain how your research adds to, or contradicts, or modifies the relevant body of knowledge. It is not just a matter of summarizing all that you have read since the beginning of your candidature. You will use the literature review to show a very direct relationship with your own research and that of others, and how this informs your own research design.

This is the first part of what a literature review does; it identifies existing knowledge and shows how your research is informed by it. Indeed, this idea of it *informing* your research is the very word that you will use. The second function of a literature review is to identify gaps in the existing literature. These gaps indicate a lack of attention by scholars, areas that are still to be examined in scholarly ways. There are many gaps within any given body of literature in any given field, gaps which provide you with openings for your own research. Having a gap in the literature, though, does not of and by itself justify the need for research in that area. You will make a scholarly case for your addressing what you have identified as being lacking. There are ways of phrasing this, such as the following:

> *This gap I have identified in the literature is one that my research has addressed. In doing so, my research will contribute to new knowledge about this field of study. At present, there is a lack of research-based material upon which to draw, so that practice in this tends to rely on belief and assumption rather than empirical knowledge. I anticipate that my research will provide research-based material upon which scholars and practitioners may draw to inform professional debate and discussion.*

Use this two-pronged feature of the literature review to focus the reading that you are doing to help you manage the task. When you do will find that you are able to narrow the reading to those areas that pertain more directly to your own area of study. Maintain a position of a focus on the reading that pertains directly to your research, not every related aspect of it.

First person pronouns and active voice

You will notice that in this example that first person pronouns (*I*, *my*) and active voice (*I have identified* rather than *has been identified*) are used. In this case, it is a matter of taking up issues related to validity and suggestions of trustworthiness discussed in the work of such scholars as Lather (1986, 1993) and Scheurich (1997). They raise issues of false impressions of objectivity in interpretivist and qualitative research when the third person pronoun and passive voice are used. You would not wish to give such false impressions in relation to ways in which you have conducted your research, and ways in which you are writing about it, as an interpretivist and qualitative researcher. Drawing on scholarly works, you will probably have made a deliberate decision to use first person pronouns and active voice. It is also possible that you have not, or that your supervisors(s) are not comfortable about your doing this. You will make your own decision on this point. Suffice to say that we prefer a frank acknowledgment of ways in which you position yourself as a researcher, so we prefer first person pronouns and active voice.

Generating the reading of the literature

You will not be alone in finding the place to start. For any of us, unless we already know the field and the major scholars working in it, most of the names of the major players in your field will mean very little. We do not necessarily know those who might be considered gurus in the field, and we generally need advice. Your supervisor(s) will guide you toward germinal works in the form of scholarly articles, research publications, publicly debated issues, as well as books and chapters in books. If you are with a well-known scholar in the field, you will consult the work that your supervisor has published as well. Indeed, it is part of the conventions of PhD writing that you cite the work(s) of your supervisor(s), so this is an important consideration for you.

The scholars whose work you consult will refer to others in the field. Read through their bibliographies and reference lists as well to see who else has been giving serious consideration to these issues in which you are interested. Use your supervisor(s) as a resource. Read the book reviews in the journal(s) relevant to your research field for more clues on who is working on what. This will enable you to engage the debate in your field. We do not operate in a world of right answers. People do not agree; they do not remain consistent. They are swayed, fashions change, new ideas emerge for consideration, and so on. Follow the debate and see how it moves across periods/eras/stages. Apart from fascinating you, it will enable you to generate a wider understanding than you will ever use in the literature review, but it will show in the confident way in which you write about the material that you do select.

At the same time, don't just rely on the reading that your supervisor(s) may suggest. Generate some searches of your own using the KEYWORDS function in going through library catalogues and databases of journals. Discuss what you have been reading with your supervisor(s). Tell them about a great article/chapter/book you've come across and recommend it to them to generate some positive discussion. Making it a two-way street makes it a lot easier, and you grow in confidence as you recommend some really important and exciting material that you have come across. You don't need to read whole books; get savvy with Contents and Index sections. Use the Library databases and the Internet to scan the abstracts of possibly useful articles, and remember that your own focus is the guiding element in all of this. You may read many works, and you will not use them all, but you will be making some important decisions about what to select for review and what not.

An annotated example

The following is a truncated copy of a PhD candidate's literature review and reference list that one of the examiners described as one of the best he had ever read. It is adapted and printed with the kind permission of the then PhD candidate.

The literature on distance education tends to be somewhat restricted to its field alone, and I turn to it before I consider the wider applications of this discussion to my own research. As matters of nomenclature, definition and characteristics are dealt with, it is necessary to examine these to inform my own practice as another researcher in the field. Keegan (1990, pp. 3–4) describes distance education as 'the Cinderella of the education spectrum' which is 'either ignored in educational journals and textbooks, in educational philosophy, educational administration or analyses of didactic technique' and even as 'an unwanted competitor in harsh fiscal times'. Indeed, he sees this lack as reflecting the absence of a firmly-based theory of distance education which would 'provide the touchstone against which decisions—political, financial, educational and social—can be taken with confidence' (p. 5). I refer to this as I have similarly found a lack of the sort of material to which he refers. This does suggest, though, a certain dynamic activity in the area of distance education as so much of the material is still in the form of journal articles and edited books, not yet in the more permanent form of bound texts and references to guide the modern practitioner or to suggest the solidity of an accepted and established mode of education. In his time in government, the Australian politician Beazley (1992, p. 5) pointed to the university 'resistance' to the inclusion of distance education mode as part of their offerings, 'related in part to a point of view that students gain a benefit from experiencing a particular kind of campus life', which immediately put them in a position of negating the 'equally valuable, if different experience of higher education' that off-campus students have. He further argued that 'Just what it is that non-attending students are missing out on is often alleged but less often demonstrated'. Somewhat predictably for a government Minister, he is concerned with the cost-effectiveness of this type of higher education access, but he does assert that in relation to the acquisition of a degree, 'there is simply no degree course in which it would be impossible to offer at least a reasonable proportion of the curriculum in this way' (p. 6). This sort of discussion does open up a range of possibilities in a globalising world for such practice. It would suggest that has the potential to move right in from the margins to occupy a central position in the educational discourse of the present times. Brown and Brown (1994, p. 31) have no doubt of this as they argue, 'Globally the literature is emphatic in pointing out that emerging technologies, particularly those involving a telecommunications component, have the potential to catapult distance learning to the forefront of the educational scene… consensus is that the new and emerging technologies hold much promise as a means to attack the enormous task of education, training and retraining facing the world as we hurtle through the few years remaining before being thrust into the twenty-first century'.

> The very first sentence is made pertinent to general considerations in relation to their own research

> The second sentence reinforces that idea of relatedness to own research before details of authors' work

> Major scholar in the field's idea given

> Something else in the literature that corroborates what's being said by and about Keegan

> Comment on perspective of this player in the field

> Says what is in the literature from other sources, always commenting on it re own research

> This is how the paragraphs work, starting on an issue of major concern in the field (minor issues not covered minor here; that belongs later in the review). Candidate is summarising, paraphrasing, quoting where it's more appropriate to do so, but keeping the variety going because it's more interesting to read than a series of quotes, and besides, a stack of quotes can be read as you trying to cover up the fact that you don't understand a particularly curly aspect of the field.

Keegan sees distance education as a 'coherent and distinct field of educational endeavour' which can provide 'a complete educational program for children and adults outside of and distinct from conventional, oral, group-based provision' by virtue of 'its own laws of didactical structures and its own quasi-industrial administrative procedures' (p. 6). He does not use the terms 'open education' and 'distance education' synonymously, seeing the open education aspect as really an administrative factor applicable to any mode of delivery. The distance factor he sees as relevant to the separation of the teacher and the learner, which therefore 'shatters the interpersonal communication of face-to-face provision' of teacher to student in traditional mode and replaces it with some form of electronic communication: print, phone, teleconference, audio, video, broadcasting, computer. Like Peters (1983, 1989), Keegan takes some time to tease out the various defining characteristic of distance education in relation to the separation, the type of administration, the student support systems and the technological media used and so on to establish the concept of a different area of educational activity, a field in which scholars may operate to build a solid theoretical base to inform the best practice possible in this area of 'quasi-permanent separation of teacher and learner throughout the learning process' (p. 44).

> Candidate makes rather confident generalisations about the style of the writing encountered. They would have had to have read a great deal of the literature before they could make so confident a comment on the literature in their review of it

The writers in this field tend to be cataloguers, developing lists of distinguishing characteristics and practices for discussion. Much of the literature reflects this attitude, concentrating rather on morphology and/or instances of practice manifesting in catalogues and lists of what is and what is not, or should or should not be considered as distance education. Moore (1993) as far back as 1971 drew a distinction between open and distance education, with the former characterised by the removal of restrictions, exclusions and privileges on the mode and method of program delivery, pointing to the unrealistic nature of such an undertaking with students then being freed from such things as entry requirements (RPL or recognition of Prior Learning he suggests as a possible substitute for candidature qualification), established academic calendars for the timing of entry to or exit from a program, and so on. In another catalogue, he establishes three types of interaction characteristic of effective learning—learner-context, learner-instructor, learner-learner, then applies their relevance to the distance education context. He sees the interaction between the learner and the content of the course as 'the defining characteristic' of education, regardless of its form or mode, that actually results in changes in the learner's understanding, and this as an essential aspect of learning regardless of mode of delivery. He does see, though, the potential for learner-learner interaction as being plumbed for a more extended learning experience that more traditional forms of education tend to ignore. The electronic-based learning groups established as part of distance education programs he sees as being a great facilitator of this (p. 200), and he introduces the idea of transactional distance as a descriptor of the distance between the student and the teacher. With Kearsley (Moore and Kearsley, 1996, p. 200), he introduces the idea of transactional

> You will make similar confident comments on the literature when you have read so much that you realise that you are not getting anything new, that the germinal works tend to cite other germinal works and rework old ground

You will be able to make such statements with absolute confidence born of being well read in the field, as opposed to the presumptuousness that we sometimes feel when we are new to the field and are overawed by the great minds who have given so much of their work to us

Signposting and linking sentence

distance as a descriptor of the distance between the student and the teacher, that is, a pedagogical distance which, while born of geographic separation, creates a 'psychological space of potential misunderstanding between the behaviours of the instructors and those of learners'. They do acknowledge that this transactional distance exists in any educational context, but say that in the distance education context it is so significant that the effects on behaviours are major ones and that therefore special organisational and teaching behaviours must be marshalled accordingly. 'How special will depend on the degree of the transactional distance', they conclude, and expand upon Holmberg's (1986) idea of the guided didactic conversation.

Moving on to next aspect of the field covered in the literature in an easy and logical manner

Candidate does not only state what has been read and noticed. That is part of it, yes, but there is another part as well. That's where they tell the examiners(s) exactly how they will use what they have read to inform their own research

Holmberg (1986, p. 2) sees distance education as a separate academic discipline. He refers to the distance factor as 'the various forms of study at all levels which are not under the continuous, immediate supervision of tutors present with their students in lecture rooms or on the same premises but which, nevertheless, benefit from the planning, guidance and tuition of a tutorial organisation'. His description of the separation is 'non-contiguous' contact. He does not see that such non-contiguity precludes personal contact as part of the separation, that such personal interaction is in fact 'the backbone' of distance education. The student, he says, is not alone in educational endeavour as tutors and supporting organisations are in place to facilitate learning through a kind of conversation, 'guided didactic conversation' to be precise (p. 4). He argues that the style of materials presentation is based on a less formal, reasonably colloquial style not found in textbooks—the tutor using personal pronouns such as 'I' and 'we', referring to the student as 'you' to personalise the contact—which 'stimulates activity and implies reasoning, discussing for and against, referring to students' personal experience and thus avoiding omissions in chains of thought' (p. 5). He puts the case (1993, p. 332) that this aspect of distance education is of vital importance if we are to avoid the propensity towards autocracy in self-contained courses, for otherwise students may not be led to develop as autonomous learners where they can 'share discoveries and intellectual experience' with an empathetic teacher (p. 337). Thus he sees the distance education mode being largely the responsibility of the organisation as the planning, guiding, tutoring agent rather than the teacher fulfilling this role, stressing the two-way communication process involved in all teaching and learning done in this mode. (Garrison, 1990, p. 7, does add a cautionary note to this emphasis on the teaching function of the organisation as he reminds us that organisations do not teach—teachers do!). Paul (1990, p. 22) also sees distance education universities as 'knowledge institutions in a knowledge society', thereby taking steps towards the appropriation of the discourse of the post-industrial reflexive society as well as the discourse of globalisation when he presents them as 'institutions which combine highly-specialised professionals with large production systems' and as organisations 'dedicated to the application of new technologies to the business of teaching and learning'. As well, he devotes some thought to the concept of open learning, considering it to be an 'elusive term

Adds interesting detail to keep the reader engaged. Takes a interactive position vis-á-vis the literature. Candidate is obviously comfortable with the exercise

(p. 40) that can only be applied as to the relative openness of a system rather than in the sense of its being open in any absolute sense, and thus more as an ideal type (p. 46) than an actual entity. His personal philosophy of education is grounded in the traditional educational discourse familiar to twentieth century practitioners within mass education systems. He believes that education is central to the development of a better life and a better world, that it is a continuing process of discovery and self-discovery in which most people can succeed given the opportunity and support. The goal of such formal learning systems is to assist people to become self-directed and independent learners in an active as opposed to a passive process. He sees true learning as leading to change and self-actualisation, and he asserts that there are many ways to learn and to teach, as there are different ways in which people learn for different knowledges and different tasks. While I will use the descriptions of processes and procedures outlined by the above writers as important informing sources for my own research into the mode of distance education, it is this last point of Paul's (1990) of which I will be most cognisant. In this, he could be establishing a credo of education in the late twentieth century. What he says on this point is not simply applicable to distance mode, or to a particular level of education, but education as a whole. What is more, in the course of his discussion he posits an essential point of difference between knowledge as a process and knowledge as a commodity (p. 83), a point I would consider as of absolute importance in my research in the context of the globalisation debate...

> Maintaining the position of keeping what is said about the literature relevant to own research

> Candidate uses it to open up another corner of the field of their own research, where they wanted to lead into a discussion of the literature on globalisation theory

> Concluding statement clearly still on track

My research will go some way towards examining just how correct such an assumption would be, tracking the possible matches between the literature descriptions of what distance education and the distance learner are and the changes that have occurred in XXX university practice as exemplified by its policy statements and their impact on their education activities over the same time.

References and citations given according to that university's requirements.

The annotated example as a model

Once you've got the hang of paraphrasing, quoting, and commenting on the literature in relation to your own research, it's a matter of staying on that track. You will give a brief summary of each reading, which you can paraphrase. It is better to paraphrase than quote unless those particular words are essential in making a point. Anybody can put together a series of quotes...there is no real challenge in that, but where you do quote, acknowledge all sources and quotations correctly...what is a real skill is being able to give a critical evaluation of each piece of the literature to which you refer. Explain the implications (issues/problems/questions/social/political/cultural and so on) of each reading in general, but don't present it as a list. Group various perspectives in paragraphs devoted to particular points to be raised. Most importantly, explain how the readings have helped you to understand issues in relation to your research. You will say quite explicitly how the literature has helped you think about issues/questions/problems/advantages/disadvantages in the design of your research in your area of investigation.

You will maintain your position as a reviewer of the literature, being careful not to let the expository essay style creep into what you are writing. What you do is generate a series of statements that appear throughout your writing at the beginning, in the middle and at the end. They serve to bring you back to the point of the literature review all the time, constantly reminding the examiner(s), and you, of the reason you are referring to the literature in the way that you are, thereby complying with the requirements of a literature review. For this reason, you will not decide to use any aspect of the literature you have read in your literature review without asking yourself the question of why you are using it, in relation to your own research project. If you can't answer this question, don't use it.

Tensions within the literature

This does not mean that you will use only that which will support your own research, for there are opposing views to be taken into consideration as well in the debate in your own area of investigation. If your answer is along the lines of: "I am using this to show how others have considered the question, but have not found that it is relevant to the way I am approaching the question," then write something along those lines. If your answer is along the lines of: "I am using this to show that I have read it, my supervisor(s) will be impressed to see how widely I have read," discard it at once. It is not relevant to your research. There may be the temptation to do this, for you will have read so much you may want to show off a little. This is a temptation that you really must resist. Select only that which is relevant to your work and don't be dissatisfied with that. Use it all to show how it sits in relation to your work.

The body of the literature review

We have established that is not enough to list all that you have read, but that you also need to consider how to group the material under relevant categories. Your literature review will tend to focus on relevant paragraphs on historical background, including classic texts, current mainstream versus alternative theoretical or ideological viewpoints, including different theoretical assumptions, different political outlooks, and other conflicts, possible approaches to the subject (empirical, philosophical, historical, postmodernist, and so on), definitions in use, current research studies, current outcomes of research about the topic, principal questions that are being asked, general conclusions that are being drawn, and methodologies and methods in use. It will not be the same as an annotated bibliography where each work is treated separately and in turn. Your skill as a synthesizing writer will come into play here.

Tense

This can get a little complicated if you use present as well as past tenses, especially as you get into a large document like a thesis. Some scholars use a convention of referring to work more than 30 years old using past tenses, and anything less than 30 years old using present tenses. Our experience is that people simply don't remember what rule they are using for when to write about someone's work in past tense and when to use present tenses. We advise that you consistently write in present tenses. Even in casual conversation people will tell you, "The Bible *says*..." Of note is the fact that the Bible is many years old, but is still being referred to in the present tense. It is just easier if you use present tenses in your review of the literature as well.

Using helpful software and friends

Having early in the piece mastered the bibliographic software that you will use, get into the habit of entering the bibliographical data (and notes, if you use that function) as you go, to save you hours of work. You may also find useful information if you are one of those who uses social media. There are very useful list-serves, blogs, Facebook, Twitter, and a plethora of other sites to ask about particularly useful literature.

The words used

- In a literature review you will find yourself constantly referring to an author or authors who *say/says*, or *state/states*, or *argue/argues* something.
- You will use phrases to refer to the role that the particular features or items from the literature play in relation to your own research like: *to inform my research*; *to support my argument that...*; *to structure the research design*, and so on.

Words not to be used

There are also words that you will use over and over in your research writing, and they may come to seem too repetitive to you so you try out different ones. This is not a problem, even if you feel they are overused words in your work. Resist the temptation to use others like the following:

- *mentions*: When someone has written a book, chapter, or article to present an argument, to suggest that they *mention* something really trivializes the work, and that is not the meaning that you want. Do not use the word.

- *posits*: One does not just *posit*. One posits something, like an idea or a suggestion, so your expression needs to be something like *Smith et al posit the idea that....* You will not write something like *Smith et al. posit that*, for this is incorrect.
- *hypothesises*: We do not work with hypotheses in qualitative research, so drop this word from your research vocabulary as well.

Stick with *says, states*, and *argues* and *posits the idea that....*

Suggested reading

There are some books on the subject, but the various handbooks and guides we have listed so far generally have a chapter on the literature review. A search to find listings of journal articles that deal with the literature review in your field will throw up quite a few such specifically focused publications.

Cooper's (1989) *Integrating research: A guide for literature reviews* is an older publication, but it is a good resource.

Hart's (2001) *Doing a literature search: A comprehensive guide for the social sciences* has a comprehensive and practical approach to identifying sources of literature for use.

Ridley's (2012) *The literature review: A step-by/step guide for students* is written in a most accessible style, with a similar approach to that of Hart.

Conclusion

You will do a great deal of reading over the next few years, all of it focused in some way. The literature review refers to a particular type of literature, the research literature in your field, and positions you as a researcher in that field. Your literature review tells a lot about you, all of it important. The other reading that you will do will be the literature search in the fields of methodology, method, technique, data analysis, and so on. You will draw heavily on that literature too, but not in the same ways as you have in this literature review chapter.

Hot Tip 4

You will read so much more than you will be able to use in this literature review, but as you start to look about for other openings for your activities as a researcher, you'll probably be able to use it most effectively in a paper you're writing for a related but differently focused conference or journal. When you do find such openings make sure that you follow up on them. These may be refereed or professional journal articles (especially on the way in which you are using methodology and method), calls for papers for special editions of journals, calls for chapters in an edited scholarly book, particular conferences in your field at which you can present your research as a Work in Progress, and so on (see also "Milestone 12: Publishing from the work.")

Milestone 5: Methodology

5

In reaching this milestone, you will be addressing the *philosophy* part of your Doctor of Philosophy. The word *methodology* is based on the Greek words *metá* (with, after), *hódos* (the way)—sometimes combined as *méthodos* (a following after)—and *lógos* (reason, account, reckoning). Given this, research methodology can be understood as the reasoning that informs particular ways of doing research, or the principles that inform the organization of research activity. Associated words that also involve this concept of a system of principles for guidance include *philosophy* (Greek: *philos*—a system of wisdom) and *ideology* (Greek: *ideo*—a combination of ideas; *idéa*—opinion, view, belief). Researchers refer to their methodology as the conceptual underpinnings or the assumptions that guide their research, as it is a theory of producing knowledge through research and provides a rationale for the way a researcher proceeds.

Methodology, in its common usage, refers to the logical assumptions that underpin research practice. The term *methodology* is used here to refer to the philosophical underpinnings that inform a given research practice. The chapter that you write on methodology is your discussion first of the theory upon which your research is based… and you will show that you understand it well… and then where you will show just how this theory applies to the research that you are doing. You will do this in quite specific ways. It is where you will show the examiner(s) that you get it. You will engage another body of literature when you write this chapter; it is the body of literature on research methodology. It is a different body of literature from the one that you engaged when reading the research literature. You will also paraphrase, quote, and cite this literature, and again, you will never make a claim about methodology that is not supported by what is in the literature on methodology. Unsupported claims are assertions, of no use to you whatsoever.

Getting the methodology

The decisions that you make in relation to methodology are important because methodology influences the research questions you ask, the type of research you do, the method and mode of analysis you use, what you extrapolate from your data, and your claims to intellectual authority. There is no universal agreement on what researchers mean by methodology. This should not be surprising; researchers are much like other people in that they often have different perspectives on the same events or issues and different interpretations of the same word(s) and/or similar concepts. What we canvass in relation to this milestone are just some among many ways in which concepts such as *research* and *methodology* can be understood. Not all researchers, including your supervisor(s), will necessarily agree on elements of methodology.

An understanding of methodological orientations will enable you to engage in scholarly debates across and within disciplinary areas. It will also help you to evolve beyond a commonsense approach to your research problem and to read, write, and think and practise at a deeper conceptual level. Your peers in the research field would also anticipate that your awareness of the complexity of methodological issues would lead to a tolerance of all approaches to research, and an appreciation of the value each has to offer.

Given the number of methodologies available for your selection, you will be expected to give some serious consideration to them, selecting from the range of options that which is most suitable to your research. It is worth noting that the methodology applies to your research, not to you. You may be using Symbolic Interactionism as your methodology, but you will not describe yourself as a symbolic interactionist, for the thesis is about your research, not you. Your methodology will necessarily result from decisions that you make regarding the manner in which data are to be gathered and interpreted, certainly, but more than this, it will result from your own stance as a researcher that results from an investigation of the research field that will underpin the decisions that you make. Your ontological and epistemological stance will take you into the possibilities suggested by theory, which is your methodology.

It is important to remember that there are no uncontested, final answers to the big methodological questions. In this book, we do not discuss in detail the many approaches to research that researchers use. We do, though, give a brief account of some approaches that will help you to understand methodologies.

A poststructuralist approach will draw on a number of theorists who give consideration to ways in which discourses construct what can be known all the while paying detailed attention to the language in which this is couched. We may refer to them as critical theorists, even if we do not apply such a term to ourselves. Critical theorists draw on Marxism as representations of ways in which the most powerful gain social, economic, and political influence, especially over the less powerful. Feminist theorists (also referred to as such, even if we are not describing ourselves in this way, and poststructuralists, and so on) can take any of these approaches but have females as the central concern of their research. The research question(s) will suggest the most appropriate methodology for you to use as you address it or them. None is superior or inferior to another; it is a matter of making a researcher's decision on what is most appropriate for the project in hand.

Poststructuralism

You may find that poststructuralism and postmodernism tend to be used interchangeably in some of the material that you encounter, but we do not do this. Postmodernism, as far as we are concerned, concerns itself with the whole world of the latter part of the twentieth century and up to our own time with its art, architecture, writing, design, and so on. We are engaging in intellectual and academic pursuits, the philosophical and theoretical issues of that postmodern world…we are drawing on poststructuralism. Artists may be postmodernists; PhD candidates who take up the theoretical positions possible in a postmodern sense are drawing on poststructuralism. There is scholarly debate on this sort of distinction between the two, but unless your research question specifically addresses this sort of debate, your thesis is not the place to pursue the discussion to any great depth beyond an acknowledgement that scholars are talking about it. Given this, we will not refer to postmodernism again.

Poststructuralism views the material world as made up of structured contradictions, that is, not coincidental or accidental ones. It sees the exploitation of such a world which can be objectively known only by removing tacit and unquestioned, taken-for-granted ideological biases. A poststructuralist approach means searching for disguised contradictions, disguised because they are hidden by ideology. As the research proceeds on these bases, spaces open up for previously silenced voices. The language that is used is specifically designated as *discourses*. We have focussed on the work of Foucault, Derrida, and Lyotard because they are considered as the scholars who produced the germinal texts upon which poststructuralism is built. There are many others, and you will encounter them in your reviews of literature as you proceed.

Discourses

The concept of discourses is integral to poststructuralist research. Discourses are social practices, not just verbal or written texts, that constitute and are constituting of a social self. The argument is that human beings do not create unified social theories or observe an objective reality, but through discourses construct and constitute their social reality. Discourses indicate not only who can speak, but also what can be said or thought, at what time or place, and with what authority. In such ways discourses constrain the possibilities of thought, keeping the unthinkable, a concept with which humans are so familiar, well and truly at arm's length. In such ways too are power relationships embodied. The social context of this has profound implications for the researcher drawing on poststructuralism, as discourses are part of processes designed to produce a docile population in the face of the power of the state. Making visible ways in which that power operates enables challenges to those mechanisms. The knowledge brought to oppressed or marginalized populations is designed to effect social change based on change and reform of institutionalized and institutional practice, and hence betterment of humanity.

Ideology

This is another concept integral to poststructuralism (and other methodologies as well, of course). Ideology represents the world in certain ways and those ways represent the interests of those in control of a socio-political system. A capitalist ideology constructs the world in the interests of those with capital so that they may ensure private rather than public ownership of the means of production of goods and services that they may sell or trade for profit in a market economy. Those who subscribe to this ideology are not all private owners of production; they are also the workers who receive their wages via this system. Capitalist ideology constructs the world as one large market of production, profit, and loss. A socialist ideology constructs the world as representing the economic interests of workers, who will own the means of production where this production will generate social rather than private wealth. Ideology constructs class, economies, and ways of life associated with it. The point of difference between ideology and theory is that ideology is based on beliefs that are not necessarily supported by any evidence. Certain beliefs about teaching, or health care, for example, are based on ideological stances. Theory is based on empirical evidence that is generally accepted in the research community, and while future research may provide evidence that will bring a given theory into question, at this time it is accepted and acceptable for a researcher's use.

Multiple perspectives

All of this would suggest that observable behavior is multiple and negotiated by and for humans through a multiplicity of processes. The researcher, to aspire to a full understanding of human behavior, will investigate the social rules which underpin it. This puts the researcher in the social picture as well, of course, as another social actor negotiating the rules which govern human behavior. The positivist ideal cannot hold here for either the researcher or the researched. Given this, we take an interpretivist position to investigate people's perceptions and everyday experience of the world as being based on mutual knowledge, largely tacit but constantly used and modified by social actors as they interact with each other. The researcher will produce accounts of their actions and those of others where the routine, taken-for-granted, unreflective attitude in which everyday life is conducted may never be consciously articulated, but in the course of poststructuralist research processes and procedures consciously construct meanings and interpretations. It is at this point that the researcher introduces procedures which encourage such reflections to discover meanings. The descriptions provided by participants in the research then become data which, when analyzed, become the technical descriptions that the researcher constructs.

Critical theorists

Research based on critical theory is a largely twentieth-century phenomenon and has its roots in the social upheavals of the 1917 Revolution in Russia which produced the first communist state the world has ever seen. The only other comparable social revolution is that of the establishment of the first democratic state in the United States after 1776. Both have been truly dramatic and radical political positions in the contexts of their times. Both have generated a number of similar political structures in other nations, and both have had profound effects on the thinking of educators around the world. The term, *critical*, in this context is not necessarily a negative concept, but one of informed appraisal of particular phenomena. In this case, it is one based on a particular form of questioning that may throw up alternative answers and/or ideas to those that are accepted or taken-for-granted without any real consideration.

Research as a political act

Critical theory sees social enquiry as a political act. Text is not the main focus here, discourse is. The critical theorists, most closely associated with Habermas (1979) base their approach on the development of liberationist theory aimed at emancipation from oppression through articulated, critiqued, and re-evaluated social experience on the part of researcher and researched, who they consider indivisible. The aim is to improve the quality of human life, not merely understanding the underpinnings of that life, or controlling it on the basis of the knowledge gleaned, or predicting outcomes of social control. They take the position that there is no validity in knowledge for its own sake; it is valid only when translated into social emancipatory action. Critical theorists do not attempt a value-free research paradigm, not only because it is an impossible stance for them to maintain but also because they see the importance of ideology, value, and belief systems in reforming their own practice, especially as these relate to issues of equity.

Critical theory constantly questions with a view to generating responses that may lead to a more just society, recognizing the power of different kinds of knowledge to shape life chances, and engaging what it sees as dialogical processes through such questioning to address real problems of real people about real lives as they live them. It recognizes that social constructs are NEVER neutral, regardless of various institutions' attempts to present themselves as such. Critical theory constructs socially constructed organizations as serving the interests of specific groups, thereby alienating others from opportunities that may improve their position in society. It concerns itself with the interests of the least powerful in a society and improving lives through raising consciousness and critique.

Feminist theorists

In similar vein, feminism takes issue with the social world constructed by men as *natural*, received as such by women, and questioned by no-one. It tackles the ontological stance based on men's ways of viewing the world, that is, an androcentric perspective which at best distorts and at worst omits women's experience of the world. The argument is that if what counts as knowledge is based only on part of humanity's experience, men's, then it can only be partial knowledge as masculine experience as understood by men and thus a distortion of human social life and thought (Weedon, 1988). It too takes the line that the knowledge generated by this type of research is valid only in its ability to transform current understandings and behaviors. It proceeds from its questioning of what constitutes reality, what is accepted as the *natural* state of the social world (for example, is biology destiny?) and thus enabling, and empowering, the forces of change.

Foucault, Derrida, Lyotard

Poststructuralist approaches may be similarly informed as the critical theorists, but by French scholars such as Foucault, Derrida, and Lyotard. They will approach discourses as exploring the possibilities of power–knowledge relationships, not as dualities or even as dichotomies, for poststructuralism posits the interrelatedness of the two. The aim is the exposure of power relations and the contribution of marginalized knowledge systems (and part of the social power relations) in the makeup of social relations. Knowledge, then, does not exist in absolute or relative terms, is far from value-free, is distorted by the very forces that generated it to serve the interests of dominant groups, and the French poststructuralists focus their attention accordingly. Power relations are in the language, where discourses name and frame subjectivities. The different inflection at the end of the two words, *feminine* and *feminist*, for example, can empower at the same time as it oppresses. Central to their thinking is the power–knowledge nexus: knowledge is power; power is knowledge.

It is possible for the poststructuralist researcher to prise taken-for-granted aspects of discourses out into the open, to challenge human understanding of power and power relations. All social sites then become sites of contestation, especially along the lines established by racism, sexism, ageism, classism, or any other sort of minority group status or identification.

Reconstructionism

Reconstructionism provides a theoretical perspective that applies to education in general and curriculum in particular. It is a challenge to the *status quo* of a given society, a challenge designed to realize an improvement of life in that society. Reconstructionism dominates developing countries' approaches to education, where the concept of education for education's sake is a luxury such countries simply cannot afford. It presumes that education benefits will flow to the rest of society, where such benefits include desired and desirable attitudes in the citizenry. Social engineering, then, is a large part of the focus. Integral to a reconstructionist position, quite different from that of reproduction, is education to achieve change by transforming curriculum. In doing this, reconstructionism looks to education systems as tools to be used in the building of new political, economic, and social orders, in particular, ones that are perceived to be better than existing or older ones. Such new social orders would be based on social concerns and having the economic structures necessary to maintain democratic systems, rather than elitist and systematic enfeeblement of nonelites. But schools are not the only social tools available to teach people; there are theater and film productions, promotions and publicity campaigns, genres of literature, and so on, any or all of which may serve as vehicles for community education programs with reconstructionist foci.

Social focus

Reconstructionism assumes that a given society has problems and identifies those problems as things like social injustice and inequality. This goes well beyond an acknowledgement of the importance of education for the good of the nation, such as announced by British Prime Minister Blair (2001) for Britain: "Our top priority was, is and always will be education, education, education," estimable as such sentiments are. It is an entire education system geared toward teaching and learning the skills and knowledge required to identify and ameliorate problems of society, where the teacher is an agent of change and reform, and the student learns to reform and reconstruct society. There is a whole world outside the classroom that may be harnessed in the service of education to build of more just society—street gangs, health services, children's and young adult literature, counseling, and so on—and researchers may use reconstructionism to focus their investigation.

Phenomenology

Phenomenology concerns itself with ways in which humans interact with the world of phenomena. These phenomena may be actions; they may be an activity; they may be relationships; they may be empirical objects. The individual who is somehow involved with the phenomenon, who experiences it in daily life, gives meaning to the phenomenon, the experience of it, and does so intentionally, even if tacitly. Van Manen (1990) points out that knowing is not just a cognitive act; one may become knowing through an inseparable connection to the world, through what it means to be human. Descriptions of what are described as "lifeworlds" are collected by lived experience and recollect lived experience, giving rise to a "validating circle of enquiry" which is "validated by lived experience and it validates lived experience." There are four elements to these lifeworlds of people: lived time, lived self, lived space, and lived other, not necessarily in that order, and not necessarily linear. There will be overlaps of the four worlds, but they become part of lived experience. Lived experience is different from experience. Experience is what happens to a person, but lived experience is that person's reflections on it so that it is given a particular meaning for the life being lived. The researcher's role is to access that reflection, possibly through interviews, diaries, and personal accounts of some kind so that it may be analyzed.

Human experience as text

Phenomenology looks to text as a tool for generating knowledge, where the whole of human experience is to be read as text of one kind or another. The point of entry of the phenomenologist is as a reader of this text, recognizing that each text is socially constructed and always being alert to questions in relation to whose readings and/or interpretations are the correct ones. The immediate phenomena of human experience require the researcher to go beyond the observable to reach into the context of that human experience to increase understanding and imply a certain level of self-understanding. This is so of course for all subjectivity in qualitative research, but phenomenology would particularly stress the interwoven nature of human experience and human understanding, raising questions to expand the horizons of the researcher and the participants in that research. It is worth noting that they are not *subjects* of research, or *the researched*, but *participants* in the research.

Symbolic Interactionism

Symbolic interactionism provides a theoretical framework for understanding people's behavior and viewpoints, where the researcher provides descriptions of processes of human interaction. The researcher examines human behavior on the basis of the meaning individuals give to their environment; as they interpret significant symbols in their worlds. The symbols are stimuli of responses that are expressed as words in processes of interpretation. In this process of interpretation, the meanings are continuously being modified and reflected upon symbolically as individuals interact with one another. Pivotal to symbolic interactionism is the concept of people as constructors of their own actions and meanings, with the focus on individual action rather than wider social structures. Individuals construct their own social realities and perspectives of their world using responses from the environment and different sociocultural relationships with which they interact. Symbolic interactionism provides opportunities for analyzing ways in which different socializing experiences affect an individual's life cycle, the argument being that individuals do not react automatically to special stimuli, but through their own constructive processes use symbols to define their actions and meanings and so acquire values and beliefs.

Generating knowledge

The empirical world becomes the world of everyday experiences, and social reality and human behavior in symbolic interaction is conceptualized as symbolic, communicated, and subjective in both structure and content. Symbolic interactionism is a means used by a researcher to provide an understanding of how people make sense of their world, employing aspects they have developed over their individual lives in a multiplicity of contexts. They become the constructors of their own actions and meanings from their own social realities as they interact with others. Symbolic interactionism is always open to new ways of development and new concepts as it revolves around concepts of self in relation to meaningful symbols that are based in language, gestures, and objects. Literature, art, and drama immediately come to mind.

Why this and not that

It is not necessary to explain differences between various theories, but it is necessary to show that you are aware of the possibilities that are open to you as a researcher. As you do this, say why, for example, having read Habermas, you have opted for the way that Foucault has dealt with discourses. Don't judge one as superior or inferior to the other; just say why one is more relevant to the way you are approaching your research question(s) than is the other. You may find that even though your reading of the methodology literature suggests that Marxist theory has been the conceptual tool that the majority of researchers before you have used, postcolonial theory, for example, may be a more useful conceptual tool for you to use for your research. You do not have to engage in an exhaustive critique of the body of the methodology literature based on Marxism for that reason, but you will be able to point out that, given the approach that you have taken, another body of methodology literature presenting different theory suits your purposes for research better. It will also allow you to indicate that, while you have done some extensive reading in this area, you have decided not to use it for very valid reasons. That way you feel better too because a lot of what you have read is not going to waste after all…it's just showing how knowledgeable you are in relation to having read just about everything there is to read in the field.

The sort of sentence that you use here is:

> *Such concern with Marxist interpretations goes well beyond the scope of my own research, so that this aspect of the literature in the field is something that I will not be drawing on in my pursuing my own research question(s) because....*

OR

> *While I appreciate the importance of such a perspective, I have similar misgivings to those of Author A in relation to Author B's approach to the problem, and I will not be using it as part of mine because....*

OR

> *The concepts of discourse and discursive practice will be most important in informing my own research design, but I will not be taking on the suggested dimension of conscious-raising of critical theory in my research because.....*

OR

> Referring specifically to the methodology literature: *As Scheurich (1997) expresses it, 'I do not pretend to have correctly "interpreted" Foucault, but it is from my repeated readings of [his] works that I developed this new way of thinking about social and education problems that the [discourses examined in this thesis] are meant to solve or alleviate' (p. 94).*

Below is a section of a thesis that was nominated for an international *Best Thesis* award. The research is informed by poststructuralism, specifically as represented in Foucault's work.

An annotated example

> Introduces Foucault as primary source and 'regimes of truth'

> Establishes own position in relation to theory as related to power and discourses

> Introduces major concept: subjectivities and their construction through discourses

> Explains understanding of ways in which social world is sustained through discourses

I take up the notion that in seeking to understand how we come to know it is not only necessary to examine the discourses that are made available, but equally important to examine the positionality of individuals within these discourses. In doing so, I have drawn upon poststructuralist theorising analyses power relations in relation to discourses. This is based on an argument drawn from Foucault's (1980) 'regimes of truth' where he argues that discourses organise our perceptions, our ways of knowing, making some things visible and others invisible, some things true and others false. … Individuals, through learning the discursive practices of a society, position themselves within those practices in multiple ways, and develop subjectivities both in concert with and in opposition to others. This means that, although our subjectivity is constructed for us, it becomes us as we actively take up subject positions. Given this, we are only able to construct ourselves within discourses that are made available to us. But since meaning is not fixed, the availability of subject positions is always in a state of flux. If we see society as being constantly created through discursive practices then it is possible to see the power of these practices, not only to create and sustain the social world but also to see how we can change that world through the refusal of certain discourses and the generation of new ones. Given this, through the analysis of discourse, poststructuralists are able to develop their understanding of the relationship between persons and their social world (Davies 1989), which has important implications in conceptualising social change …

> Discusses link between language, knowledge, and power

> Engages concepts of normalising effects of discourses

… Within poststructuralist theories, the individual is constructed by the discourses that are available. The individual is also able to resist certain discourses, but the effects of normalisation operate so that individuals will privilege particular constructions of their subjectivity.… For Foucault (1980:93) language, knowledge and power are inextricably linked. ... This discourse is the conjunction between power and knowledge. …

> Statement summarises key points of the preceding and suggests the next concepts to be discussed

> Discursive practice defined and explained

Discourse, as a noun, refers to the way in which particular ways of speaking have been institutionalised and in such ways become constitutive of people and their actions (Davies and Harré 1991/92). Discourses are constituted by exclusions as well as inclusions, by what can be said as well as what cannot be said. The way in which individuals or groups are included or excluded functions as a normalisation. Discourse as practice, *discursive practice*, is the ways people constitute themselves and are constituted by others (Davies and Harré 1991/92). Discursive practices include the way our talk constitutes other aspects of our world, in particular the component of … nature. Subject refers to the way we think about ourselves and act; it refers to discourses and practices that pre-exist us to which we are accountable. Our subjectivity, then, is a product of discourses and practices to which we are subject, a result of particular constructions of subjectivities through discursive practices, that is, normalisation…I have argued that if we accept that normalisation is a technique which gives rise to marginal

> groups taking up hegemonic discourses, then it is possible to argue that these discourses are not imposed by 'police' restrictions, but that they seduce, manipulate and encourage normalisation. ...
>
> Foucault (1984:44) draws attention to the tension between a fixed conception of human nature and the process of critical awareness. Foucault rejects the concept of fixed human nature as he sees this as one of the practices of normalisation and homogenisation of the individual. ... For Foucault, it is this attempt to normalise and homogenise individuals through the production of 'truth' that acts against the freedom of individuals. Thus, the use of metanarratives such as the metanarrative of justice, rationality and (I assume) equality is understood to work against the 'free' postmodern self... Although I find Foucault's suggestion not to engage in normalising techniques appealing, I have not been able to identify how this might be possible in practice. Although it may be in some utopian sense a 'good' idea to avoid normalising practices, our embeddedness in the discursive practices of society and its institutions might mean that this cannot be achieved in the practical realm. Even if we choose to avoid institutions such as schools and churches, we are not freed from other forms of institutionalisation. We are born into families, we live in communities and throughout our lives we must cohabit with other members of this planet (whether human or non-human). The question for me is not whether we should endeavour to avoid relationships and hence some forms of institutionalised behaviours but, rather, can we educate future generations to question taken for granted truths, so that normalised behaviours are critiqued for their effects.

Discusses subject position and subjectivity as constructed by and constructing discourses

Returns to 'regimes of truth' as problematic

Personal response to the theory clearly articulated

Before going on to other concepts, maintains personal, scholarly engagement with what is here

References and citations given in the style required by that university.

The annotated example as a model

This candidate has started their discussion of methodology with an explicit engagement with poststructuralism in general, and with the work of Foucault in particular. They have introduced most salient concepts, such as *regimes of truth* to set up a discussion of the inappropriateness of considering that there is any such thing as *truth* itself to be addresses, and finishes this section on that point. Having canvassed other key concepts—discourses; subjectivities; the relationship between language, power, and knowledge; normalization, and so on—the candidate shows just how their own personal positioning as a researcher comes into play and ways in which this raises particular questions for them. The point to be made here is that this not just an abstract discussion of abstract concepts; it is a discussion of abstract concepts in relation to this very concrete thing that is their research. There is very real evidence of very real engagement by the researcher with the theoretical material that they use in their research.

The words used

Words like ontology, epistemology, and methodology cannot be reduced to simple, fixed, unambiguous definitions. We can no more provide a precise three-line definition of epistemology than of everyday words like love or justice—these are terms that will always be the subject of exploration, speculation, and debate. You will go into some detail in your discussion of these in your thesis.

- *In making my decisions regarding selection of methodology, I have taken up the idea of relative applicability of theories suggested by Mathews (1989). He suggests that, depending on what is required in and of research, one theory may be more applicable than another.*
- *I argue that it is possible to imagine and develop a nonpositivist science if we look to understanding the social aspects of the world, including environment, and applying relevant methodologies as tools to enhance that understanding.*
- *[Poststructuralism/Phenomenology/Symbolic Interactionism...*insert relevant words here*] provides a powerful tool to underpin research and I have turned to it to inform the design of the research and the analysis of the data generated.*
- *The concept of discourses enables the researcher to make visible ways in which language names and frames subjectivities, and I have drawn on this as a powerful research tool to examine....*
- *I have examined various methodologies available to me in the research endeavor and argue that poststructuralist theories provided me with the tools to explore issues relating to the unequal power relations between .... and ... ways of knowing and also a way to examine the power relations between particular...*
- *I have drawn on the concept of discourses as constituted by and being constitutive of individuals, which provide the tools to reconstruct and deconstruct discourses of...*
- *Poststructuralist theory offers me tools to explore not only questions of who exercises power, and the practical outcomes of exercising this power, but also how the mutual constitution of individuals is achieved.*

Words not to be used

- *asserts*: This means that a claim is being made without anything evidence or data being offered to support it. We do not work with assertions at all, so don't use it.
- *believes*: This is worse than *asserts* for belief need have no basis in fact at all. Drop this word in your research writing.
- *true or truth*: We are not looking to establish any sort of truth. Indeed, if you are taking a poststructuralist position, the idea of truth is highly questionable. You only need to discuss the concept of *regimes of truth* in order to dispose of any suggestions that *truth* is a feature of your research. It is another word you will not use.
- *mankind, he/him, seminal,* and so on: This is sexist language that we do not use in our research writing. We use *humankind*, the more general *they/them* and *germinal* and so on. Some of the material to which we refer will use sexist language, and we can cite it and use [*sic*] to indicate that we understand that this is not quite correct, but that that's the way it is in the original text. It may become tedious, both for you and the examiner(s) so the first time that you encounter it, or use an example of it in your thesis, put in a footnote, something like: *I do not endorse this sort of sexist language, but rather than putting* [sic] *in repeatedly, I acknowledge its inappropriateness here.*

Suggested reading

The handbook and guides that you have consulted on general research methodology will guide you to more specific scholars in various fields.
Thomas Kuhn's (1970). *The structure of scientific revolutions* gives an excellent critique of established research paradigms that you may use to make a scholarly case for proceeding the way that you propose.
The books by Habermas, Weedon, Foucault, Derrida, and Lyotard are essential reading for you if you are working in these areas.
Denzin's (1992) work, *Symbolic interactionism and cultural studies* is a work that is well worth consulting on this topic.
If you turn to phenomenology you will use most of the material written on this by Max van Manen.
The book that we all consult at this stage of our progress is that of Denzin and Lincoln (2000): *Handbook of qualitative research.* It is a collection of detailed and sophisticated discussions on a variety of methodologies.

Conclusion

As with the literature review milestone, the completion of the methodology chapter will have a two-pronged aspect to it. You will not only show that you have a thorough understanding of the methodology you have selected, and your reason for its selection; you will also show how this sits in relation to your research. As you do this, you will situate your research within larger conceptual frameworks, develop your research identity, develop a coherent and consistent research design, and establish intellectual credibility in your field.

You will start the chapter with a reference to your research question(s) and you will end it with a reference to your research questions, but you will also signpost the relationship in each paragraph and section of the chapter. If there is anything about the methodology that is not made relevant to your research, you will discard it because you will know yourself that it is not helping your case. You will also take great pains to ensure that you make no claims that are not supported by references to the considerable body of the literature on methodology. Unsupported claims are assertions, and, again, these are of no use to you whatsoever.

A note of caution: there is a danger of being intellectually debilitated by, or getting lost within, methodological questions. Remember: there are no uncontested, final answers to the big methodological questions. As a PhD candidate with a limited amount of time to complete your research your aim is to become knowledgeable about the methodological debates that underpin your thinking to make a sound research-based decision that you can support in scholarly fashion. One way to avoid such traps is to be consistent in the words that you use:

Methodological or theoretical *approach*
Ontological and epistemological *position*
Case study/discourse analysis/ethnography (etc.) *method*
Interview/focus group/document analysis (etc.) *technique*

Hot Tip 5

Having acted on Hot Tip 2, you now know how to use bibliographic software and have been entering your references on a weekly basis. Take a further step toward efficiency and download the Thesis Template from your word processor program, or use the one provided by your university. It is set up for the sections that have no page numbers, those that have Roman numerals, and those that have Arabic numerals. Keying your work straight into this template from the outset will save days at the end of your writing of this thesis. This will be the time when you need it most, just as you are about to submit.

Milestone 6: Method

6

New researchers or research candidates have a tendency to conflate method and methodology, and one way to keep the distinction alive in your mind and in your work is to include in your planning for writing your thesis two different chapters, *Methodology* and *Method*. Remember, methodology *provides reasons* for using method such as case study or ethnography. At the same time, it is useful to have a section headed *Technique*, such as doing a survey or interviewing research participants in your method chapter. Keeping these three to be considered separately will help to focus on what each is and does in relation to your research.

Established scholars may deliberately argue for particular methods to be considered as methodologies, and this may be confusing to you. It may be the case that they are arguing for a more advanced standing for a method with which they are particularly involved, as Yin (2014) does for case study method, for example. Do not discard the reasoning behind such arguments, for often they show a deep insight to the ramifications for a particular method, but do not get into a debate about this in your thesis either. Point out to the examiner(s) that you are aware of such arguments but that you have focused on it as method to be used in research, and in such ways maintain the distinction between method and methodology in your thesis.

Getting the method

Given this, you will maintain your position that research methods are modes or ways of conducting research, a sort of package of strategies for gathering evidence. One could reasonably argue that all evidence-gathering packages of strategies fall into one of the following three categories: listening to (or interrogating) informants or participants in the research; observing behavior; or examining historical traces and records. In this sense, there are only three methods of social inquiry, with subcategories of these. Taking a poststructuralist approach, you would select a method that allows you to generate data that may be analyzed in relation to things like deconstruction, and discourse analysis. Using phenomenology as your methodology, you may decide upon method which enables you to generate data that may be analyzed out of field work, historical analysis, participant-observation, interviews, and conversation analysis. Symbolic interactionism would possibly guide you toward methods that enable you to generate and analyze data in relation to conversation and text analysis, expansion analysis, and dialectical analysis. You may find that as you get into details of your research design that there is overlap in these, and you will make a scholarly argument, based on the method literature, for your decisions in this regard.

Possible methods

We have focussed on a relatively small number of methods, but they are the most common: case study, ethnography, document analysis, discourse analysis, and narrative enquiry. As with methodologies, it is not a matter of one of these being superior or inferior to another, but one of the method's appropriateness for your research. Again, as with the literature review and methodology chapters, you will take a two-pronged approach: you will show your thorough understanding of the method and you will show how this is relevant to your research, signposting as you go to keep you and the examiner(s) engaged in your writing about your research.

Selection of method

What method you use will largely be informed by your methodology, and when you make the scholarly argument for your selection, you will show how method is consistent with methodology in this case. The point is, as always, how this pertains to YOUR research. A given methodology does not necessarily preclude or require particular method, but while a poststructuralist approach, perhaps with a focus on Foucault, will turn to an analysis of discursive formations rather than case study, a phenomenology, and a symbolic interactionist approach may both use case study method. By the same token, each may elect to use ethnography, or narrative enquiry, and so on.

Case study

Case study is a common method used by qualitative researchers because it is consistent with interpretivism, a method that allows the researcher to focus very specifically on an instance of the field under investigation. Hakim (1987) likens the method to the intense focus of a microscope on a specimen, pointing to the value of the approach in relation to achieving "experimental isolation of selected social factors within a real-life context so as to provide a strong test of prevailing explanations or ideas" (p. 61). It is a feature of case study that you would be able to exploit in your research to generate what Stake (1995a, 1995b) calls "rich descriptions" in a "bounded study" (p. 2). Within such a bounded study, you are able to group the features under review most specifically, yet allow maximization of what is learned as far as your question in general is concerned. There is a rider to this: the scope normally offered by case study is most valuable to a phenomenology or symbolic interactionism research project. It does not have that sort of value for poststructuralism, because of poststructuralism's focus on discourses and discursive formations.

Discursive formation

A researcher taking a poststructuralist approach will not turn to case study method, but will take up the concept of discursive formations. Discursive formations are networks of discourses constructing and being constructed by subjectivities, so that the concept of a bounded study with implied limitations of contexts and situations will not work. Discursive formations open up possibilities for examining discourses and their interconnectedness as part of a power–knowledge nexus. A network of a number of discourses and the possibilities this presents for focus in constructions of subjectivities provides spaces for rich explorations. Medicine is such a discursive formation, as is law, social rites of passage, indeed anything that takes your attention in the social world. Within the identified discursive formation, it is possible to tease out for closer examination discourses of economics, regulations, laws, conventions, and taken-for-granted assumptions that make up the particular discursive field. It is not bounded as a case study is, but has threads of discourses woven throughout the formation itself.

Ethnography

Ethnography is literally *writing about people*. More broadly speaking, it is any study of a group of people for the purpose of describing their sociocultural activities and patterns. Its central aim is to understand another way of life from the point of view of the person experiencing that way of life and as such, always implies a theory of culture. Ethnography takes a step away from the sort of research that describes *subjects* and *behaviors* and focuses on *actors* and *actions*. Ethnography leads the researcher into participant-observation, where they become part of a given community, living as they do, and observing the outcome of this activity. This does not necessarily mean just studying culture or a single culture as a whole, but also particular types and sections of culture—organizational or corporate culture within a western capitalist culture, for example—the unobservable values, assumptions, beliefs, and norms constituting a particular culture as being inferred through an organization's use of concrete aspects: symbols, myths, and rites and rituals.

Ethnography operates on the basis of question-discovery, with discoveries leading to more questions as knowledge increases as a result of careful observations. Researchers using ethnography as their method constantly set themselves questions to answer in relation to protocols and processes underpinning a set of cultural resources—stocks of knowledge, routines, strategies, and so on—ways in which actors in various sites collectively negotiate and achieve social order, understandings, and working relationships. The researcher enters the culture themselves, observing and documenting a particular perspective, based on the understanding that meanings and interpretations are not fixed entities but generated through social interaction. The researcher also understands that these may change: that actors' identities are subjected to processes of *becoming* that are always ongoing rather than fixed or static. Such a process understands that identities are socially constructed and that there is no single meaning for any of them (such as a woman being at one and the same time wife/mother/sister/aunt; a man being husband/father/brother/uncle and so on). This researcher works on the basis of there being multiple and competing definitions in every social order.

Document analysis

Document analysis may also be taken as discourse analysis, taking the documents under analysis as discourses which construct and constitute their own social reality. The American Declaration of Independence, for example, famously enshrined humanity's, not just American humanity's right, to "the pursuit of happiness" in a political document. In doing so, it constructed a social reality for a United States citizenry not seen before, brought into existence in the revolutionary intellectual climate of The Enlightenment in the context of revolutionary political change. From this example, we may take it that document analysis takes into consideration the totality of the context in which the document has been generated, implemented, and ultimately evaluated.

The documents may be policy statements, edicts, legal papers, Acts of Parliament or some other legislation, editorials, newspaper and magazine articles, research reports, bills of lading for cargo ships, and so on. The researcher would analyze each of such documents as having been born of its own time and the concerns regarding their content at that time. If the researcher analyzes documents produced over an extended period or periods of time, they will look for shifts regarding attitudes, beliefs, actions, and so on, and most likely policy underpinnings and organizational requirements of what is being analyzed evolve and are put into place.

Discourse analysis

Analyses of discourses are based on the principle that everything is never said, pointing up the deficiencies of the statements themselves in that aspect. This silence is as indicative as that which is said, as this enables studies of what exists in the silence as well as what is articulated.

This is part of a distribution of discourses, of things said and things concealed in relation to the central questions: "Who is speaking, who is accorded the right to do so, who is qualified to do so, from where comes the presumption that what he [*sic*] says is true" (Foucault, 1973, p. 50). These are questions that have a direct bearing on power relations in any society. Analyses establish the privileging or foregrounding of particular discourses over any possible others, and this is more than a matter of the activities of governments, regardless of their form. Churches, courts, universities, medical centers, schools—all of these and more have their roles within considerations of discourse analysis.

Narrative enquiry

Narrative has traditionally been the preserve of literature and life stories, set apart from the world of the researcher. In spite of such traditional positioning, qualitative researchers increasingly take up the possibilities that narrative enquiry offers. Narrative enquiry offers examination of different modes of thought to support research in relation to different ways of telling about the world. It offers a dimension of examining the social world that enable data to be interpreted in new ways, through social comprehension, in effect, that make possible different telling of data generated by the researcher. These are referred to as narrative ways of knowing. Their significance for us as qualitative researchers is their capacity to lead us to an understanding that there is no one true telling of data that in narratives multiplicity of expression and understanding is left intact. Taking up this notion, those of us engaged in producing knowledge that is not reducible to a single voice or an expression of one correct analysis can find scope for our research in narrative.

Validity and trustworthiness

Issues of quality in qualitative research have increasingly attracted researchers' interest in relation to ensuring the quality of qualitative study, and you will indicate a similar interest in your discussion of questions of validity. The work of Lather (1993) and Scheurich (1997) present a basis from which qualitative researchers may address questions of validity in their research. Lather has identified validity as "a regime of truth" (p. 674) that has normalized researcher activities along lines established in positivist traditions, and one which may be challenged in interpretivist paradigms. This does not mean that issues of validity are not to be engaged, but that positivist views of validity may be challenged. Scheurich gives us the idea of what has come to be taken-for-granted positioning in regard to validity as *masks*, ones which do not at all achieve what they purport to do in relation to validity, which may preclude or distinguish the knowledge of the untrustworthy or the invalid from the rest. Such considerations suggest fertile ground for our discussions as far as issues of validity for interpretivist research is concerned.

Given this, as a qualitative researcher you will not take up notions of positivist researcher emphases on measurement and quantifiable and quantified data in an attempt to achieve objectivity, but focus on establishing trustworthiness in relation to your research. The method that you select may include a number of trustworthiness devices in your research design to establish its rigor; it becomes a matter of establishing credibility, transferability, dependability, and conformability.

Credibility is achieved by maintaining internal consistency in the design, using such strategies as researcher reflexivity. Transferability is the extent to which research outcomes are applicable in other research contexts, established by careful documentation of the research itself and its context within the wider body of research literature. Dependability is established by the researcher establishing a direct relationship between the data and the activities within a given site that generated it… they must align. Conformability takes the place of objectivity in qualitative research, for we acknowledge that research, even that conducted in positivist and quantitative style, is never objective, so we design our research to conform with protocols of interpretivist and qualitative research. Such things are taken up by the reader of the research; they are not part of an abstract set of concepts to be applied. They are features involved in a series of measures, singly or in combination, taken to address issues of bias. In employing them you will establish trustworthiness in your qualitative research, as suggested below.

Trustworthiness techniques

Triangulation

Triangulation is a foremost consideration in much qualitative research. It is an attempt to gain more than one perspective on what is being investigated. It may be two or more perspectives, despite the *tri* of *triangulation* (see this chapter for a more detailed discussion on triangulation).

Bracketing

We are indebted to Husserl (1931) for the concept of bracketing. This is a conscious and intentional intellectual device used by qualitative researchers, especially those whose methodology is phenomenology, consciously and deliberately placing themselves beyond their own constructions, preconceptions, and assumptions that may be closely related to what is being researched. It infers the trustworthiness of research work.

Reflexivity

Reflexivity is the qualitative researchers' capacity to identify ways in which their own attitudes, beliefs and positioning might influence their understandings of the meanings and contexts what it is that they are researching. An important dimension of this capacity is to step away from what they have thus identified, while acknowledging their own roles in the conduct of their research.

Emics and etics of research

Such considerations in relation to trustworthiness notwithstanding, as qualitative researchers in an interpretivist tradition, we are ourselves one of the instruments in our research. The emic view is the view from the inside. The etic view is the view from the outside. The emic and the etic views are considerations in relation to your research that establish or describe ways in which you are an insider or an outsider: perhaps as a participant in the research yourself; perhaps as an outsider looking in. In relation to your research, you will make it clear just what the distinction between the researcher and the participant is. You may find yourself showing that there is very little distinction indeed (emic) or a great deal (etic). It is a useful continuum to take into account when positioning yourself.

You may position yourself at one end or the other, in between, or on a moving scale: from outsider in or insider out, for example. In doing this, you will be rejecting that notion of the objective researcher so dear to the positivist quantitative heart that purports that there is not even a researcher at all, so objective are they. We do not follow this line, remember; we acknowledge and detail the influence that the researcher themselves and the research itself may have on the environment in which the investigation occurs.

As qualitative researchers following conventions of interpretivism, we identify the areas that had been the subject of inattention until we came across them. We design the research project itself accordingly. We identify the people, documents, phenomena, contexts, and so on, of the research. We approach people to survey and interview; we organize access to documents; we seek permission to use the personal material of others; we build relationships with the participants in our research. Not only do we not shy from these features of our research, or apologize for them, or disguise them in some way, we embrace them, acknowledge them, and detail them. Given this, when you detail such features of your research you will position yourself in some way as an insider. This is the emic and etic part of the research that you will write about, showing the examiner(s) just how involved you are.

You may be involved in particularly sensitive areas within your field, especially if these are political and economic, or on the margins of socially dominant or acceptable practices. You may have spent a good deal of time building trust between you and the participants, to the extent that it only you and no one else that could possibly access or generate the relevant data. You will make this clear.

Emic considerations also involve your personal reactions, predispositions that may be confirmed or challenged, biases, or a personal history with the participants or their organization. This is an area where your own research notebooks, research journals, research diaries are most important. At the same time, your interactions with participants, organizations, documents, and so on, may dispose you to a more observational and distant position, where your own reactions are not so entwined with what you are researching, so your etic view is what is to be commented upon.

Emic: ethnography and insider researcher

An ethnographic study suggests itself as a foremost example of emic considerations. Perhaps not as visible, but needing consideration nonetheless, is the insider researcher. A researcher may have phenomenology as the methodology, case study as the method, and participants as fellow practitioners in a given organization, but there is more to it in relation to insider. The insider researcher is actually involved with the participants as one of them, working alongside them, taking up the same goals and practices geared toward achieving them while researching these very things in which all are engaged...research. The insider researcher has a dual role, in effect, as both a participant and a researcher. This is not just a gulf between the profession and the laity, important as this is when discussing language, protocols, procedures, and conventions of a given profession. Rather than seeing this as a disadvantage, in qualitative research we take up its suggestive possibilities for our research.

An annotated example

Signposting → I have discussed issues of choosing case study as my research method ← **Defining case study method** before turning to research strategies used. Case study is an investigation with a focus on a certain aspect of a particular phenomenon to gain an understanding of its meaning in its own and possibly wider situations. Yin (2006) argues that case study may be used to tease out **Use of major scholars** → the specificity of the phenomenon selected for the research, a specificity which makes it different from other phenomena, but which may produce research outcomes from which generalisations may be made to a wider context. Merriam (1998) argues that case study is used to generate a deep understanding of contexts and meanings in relation to what is being investigated. Case study method, then, allows researchers to conduct detailed investigation of particular phenomena of interest in particular contexts (Hartley, 2004; Robert E. Stake, 1995).

Explores and explains benefits of the method → Given Yin's (2006) view of case study as being based on real life experience rather than what may occur in laboratory or clinical trials, it is a method that is appropriate in interpretivist qualitative research, such as my own. Case study as a method, as George (2006) argues, allows the researcher to conduct a detailed examination of an aspect of a phenomenon in order to develop an understanding of it as a whole. The ← **Applies benefits to own research** strength of case study lies in its focus on interactive processes within specific phenomenon to identify in some detail all that may come into play (Bell, 1993). The very specificity of detail allows for fine-grained **Details of how applied in own research** → research foci that allow the researcher to avoid the broad brush stroke approaches of other methods. In my research, I have applied that detailed focus to XXXX state, then on two regions within it, and then on six sites within those regions in order to pick up on details of XXX as they play out in individual XXXX within the larger context of the vast country that is XXX. This has allowed me to pick out details for ← **Specific reference to discussion as informing own research** focussed attention, and on the basis of these, generate a number of knowledgeable insights to [issues raised by my research questions]. According to Merriam (1998), case study focuses on studying the key features of a case — processes, contexts and discoveries — a concept on which I have drawn in designing my research

According to Yin (2006), researchers taking up case study method consider three factors: research topics, contexts and data sources. This is particularly so with regard to a focus on an investigation of **Elaboration on features of the method** → a current phenomenon in a real context (Yin, 2003a, 2003b, 2006). Hartley (2004) points out that case study 'is particularly suited to research questions which require detailed understanding of social or organizational processes because of the rich data collected in context' (p. 323). I have drawn on these perspectives to take up case study as it has allowed me to highlight major issues raised by my research question [restates research question]. This question has guided me to an emphasis on the contexts in which the XXX under study has ← **Shows how method leads to techniques for data collection** been positioned, and ways in which it has been initiated and implemented on the basis of documents, interviews and a questionnaire. Such consideration feeds into what my case study elaborates…

Annotation	Example text	Annotation
Emphasises notion of 'rich' data →	As Hartley (2004) argues, researchers use case study on the basis of rich data sources to explore the phenomenon under study in relation to detailed and complex interactions and processes that occur within a social context. … I have used case study as my research method to enable me to generate a deep understanding of what the reform under study means in the context of XXX. …	← Finishes section on specific reference to own research

Citations given in the style required by that university.

The annotated example as a model

The candidate has taken some pains to be explicit and specific in the use of case study method. They have defined it, drawing on established scholars in the field to support the argument given for using it. Not only that, the candidate has also consistently applied the claims made and the arguments given for case study method to their own research, reminding the examiner(s) of the research question being addressed and explaining ways in which what is being discussed applies to the research undertaken. The paragraphs have been carefully structured, which also gives an example of that Fairy Tale principle underpinning paragraph construction.

The words used

- *I have developed a qualitative study, using case study method to locate the specifics of the phenomenon selected, specifics which make it different from other phenomena, but which may produce research outcomes from which generalizations may be made in relation to a wider context.*
- *In conducting the discourse analysis, I have been informed by the work of Derrida (1973) on texts and their contexts. I have read the transcripts of interviews as texts without assuming that they contain meaning within themselves alone, but in the articulation and reading of them, that is, the contexts in which they are produced by participants in the research and accessed by me as the researcher.*
- *I have focused on document analysis because this has enabled me to generate a different and, in relation to the research, more complete picture that has become especially evident when identified gaps between the written forms of practice and the activities forms in procedures and protocols were matched. This then guided me to discursive practice.*
- *I have used discourse analysis not from a belief in its superiority, but because I consider it a most useful tool for the task in hand, one among a raft of such analytical tools.*
- *I have not attempted to lay claim to validity within the design of this research, having rejected this as epistemologically inappropriate. My emphasis is on discourses, where I have looked to rigorous analyses rather than opinion and belief in the design of my own research program, as well as include a range and variety of texts for analysis.*
- *My role as insider researcher has enabled me to access the research environment and have prior knowledge of the field in which my research is situated. In taking my position as insider researcher into consideration I am also aware of bias or preconceived ideas which may exist in relation to the data I have gathered through the use of questionnaires, focus group transcripts, and my professional journal extracts.*

- *I have engaged issues of trustworthiness in relation to my research by taking up issues of insider researcher, connecting these with concepts of bracketing and methods of triangulation, and taking further steps in relation to reflexivity.*

Suggested reading

Research method (specific)

1. Case Study
   Stake's (1995) *The art of case study research* is the book that you will be expected to have read if your method is case study.
   Yin's (2014) *Case study research: Design and methods* is into its fifth edition, a sure indication of its being appreciated by researchers. It is the other book on case study that you will be expected to have read. Case study method receives a good deal of attention from Yin (2003, 2006).
2. Ethnography
   Hillyard's (2010) *New frontiers in ethnography* takes you through a history of work in this field and then updates to more recent considerations in ethnography.
3. Narrative Enquiry
   Leonard and Mertova's (2007) *Using narrative inquiry as a research method: An introduction to using critical event narrative* is recommended because of its focus on providing an introduction to the method, something which may be built upon with more detailed and extended reading.
4. Discourse Analysis
   Wodak and Meyer (2009), in their *Methods for critical discourse analysis*, bring together the work of a number of important scholars in this wide field. Again, this is a good place to start.
5. To flesh out the understandings generated from your engagement with such texts, scholarly articles, chapters of edited books, conference proceedings and presentations, and so on may be accessed by careful searches of electronic data bases and Web sites.
6. A rider to this: Web sites are not part of peer review protocols...any fool can put anything on the Web. You are well advised to stay clear of such material, for it may be highly questionable. If you doubt this, try out the *flatearth.com* site.

On validity

Lather's (1986) *Issues of validity in openly ideological research: Between a rock and a soft place* is a classic reference in relation to issues of validity as she shows us how possible tensions for an interpretivist researcher may be resolved.

Scheurich's (1997) *Research method in the postmodern* gives us his suggestion of validity in association with masks. It is an invaluable resource in discussions of validity, trustworthiness, and authenticity that positions interpretivist qualitative research as beyond reproach as far as validity is concerned. Used with the Lather's paper, it may be used to make a most convincing argument.

A good place to start with emics and etics is Headland's (1990) Chapter 1 in *Emics and etics: The insider/outsider debate*.

Conclusion

Your research method is your way of proceeding in gathering the data that you will analyze in producing new knowledge. Your selection from the possibilities open to a qualitative researcher will have proceeded from your understanding of ontology, epistemology, and methodology. As you give your considerations to method, you will also consider issues of validity and emics and etics associated with this. You will have made scholarly informed decisions (that is, decisions based on the literature on method in general and your selected method in particular) and you will have argued the case for the *suitability* of the method, and not argued for its superiority or inferiority in relation to any other possible method. So far you have been focussed on largely academic work at your desk in your study, and you may be impatient to get to the nitty gritty of the actual research, following the design you have worked out, and start surveying, interviewing, classifying, and so on. Before you do, though, think about technique.

Hot Tip 6

Don't even consider getting into interviews, surveys, and so on, until you have methodology and method very firmly established in your head. As supervisors, we have too often found that candidates have ignored this advice and collected a whole lot of data that they virtually cannot use, for what they have done has not been consistent with methodology or method. This has happened because they have not been inclined in the early stages to wrestle with the complexities of the *Philosophy* part of the degree, and then found themselves rather at a loss at the later stages.

Milestone 7: Technique

7

In reaching this milestone, you have been becoming increasingly practical in engaging issues in your design of your research. In writing up your decisions and the intellectual processes through which you arrived at them, you will once again use that two-pronged feature of the previous chapters: show the examiner(s) that you understand the technique or techniques you have selected, and ways in which this relates to your research. An important practical thing to do is to trial or practise your techniques on a group of others, perhaps friends and colleagues, who will not be participants in the research itself. That way you will know what works and what does not, and those friends and colleagues may also give useful feedback on how they responded to what you were asking them to do. This is also part of your training to become doctorly in your research. Experienced researchers set up a trial run of the research instruments they intend to use, simply because it is a good idea to help anticipate potential problems and resolve any issue before the research itself is put into action.

The word *technique* comes from the Greek word *tekhne* and implies expertise or the art or craft of performing a particular task. It also implies a connection with a larger technology and signals that particular research methodologies and methods guide research techniques. Some call it data collection instrument design, or strategy, or data-generating techniques. We refer to the tools that you use to generate your data as the techniques that you use. You will probably use a number of techniques: interviews and transcripts of interviews plus field notes; focus group plus professional journal; observation plus field notes; the wording or phrasing of documents plus interviews; the items in diaries or journals plus surveys; your observation notes plus photographs plus video tapes; and so on. This is part of your efforts at triangulation which you will recall is an attempt to gain more than one perspective on what is being investigated. It may be two or more perspectives, despite the *tri* of *triangulation* (see also "Milestone 5: Methodology" chapter).

Interview

It seems simple enough to generate data on a given topic by conducting interviews…you ask questions and the person answers them. This is what we do when we interview, of course, but that is only the beginning of a complex set of factors to be considered when using interview as a technique for generating data. Formulating open-ended questions designed to elicit detailed responses is a major consideration in using this techniques. Questions that will give you *yes* or *no* answers will not take you very far in getting to the *how* and *why* of the research questions you are pursuing. You will make a video or audiotape of the interviews that you conduct, and transcribe them for close analysis.

A not inconsiderable consideration is the very fact of the audio or video recorder's presence and any possible effects this might have on the data to be gathered in this

Milestone Moments in Getting your PhD in Qualitative Research

way. The presence of a recording device is not to be seen as a neutral feature of the interactions between researcher and research participant (Thompson, 1996).

We find Block's (1995) metaphor of the taped interview as a dirty window through which some, but not all, of what may be seen is visible a most apt metaphor in relation to this. Those that you interview may have reasons of their own for not saying all that they know or have experienced about what you are asking, and they have every right to this. They may also just be plain lying to you. They may find the tape recorder itself an inhibitor to what they might say, or they may find it an irresistible impetus to hyperbole.

If you select this technique, and it is a common one in qualitative research programs, you will also include discussion of the transcription processes and procedures involved, and the ethics considerations of having tapes transcribed by someone other than yourself who is not therefore part of the research itself. Again, you will indicate how you have addressed such things.

You will engage some scholarly discussion on just how far you may go in relation to trustworthiness in the use of interviews. This does not mean that they are not to be used; what it does mean is that you demonstrate to your examiners that you are aware of what is involved, and how you have addressed this.

Focus group

The focus group is where a group of usually 8–10 people, but sometimes up to 20, are brought to a centralized place to respond to questions or a topic of particular interest to a person or an organization, conducted by a facilitator or moderator. More than 20 people means that not everybody gets to have their say, or too much material results so that it becomes unmanageable.

As with any techniques used in research, it is a complex phenomenon, especially in relation to the explicit use of group interaction to produce insights not as easily gained by other methods. The participants do not just react to the facilitator or moderator on a one-to-one basis; they react and interact with each other as they explore aspects that come up in discussion. To enable this to happen implies an important role for the moderator or facilitator. As it is a structured and purposeful conversation, not an unplanned or spontaneous dialog, the authoritative role of the focus group facilitator or moderator is vital, if the efficiency and the quality of the data gathered is not to be adversely affected. That facilitator or moderator may pick up on nonverbal signs, these being at least as significant, if not more so, as the words that are spoken, adding a valuable dimension to enriching the data.

At the same time, the moderator is to ensure the nonthreatening environment in which a free and frank interchange of views is to occur. This does require some preparation, based on a clear understanding of what and how discussion is to occur. Toward the end, the moderator will draw the session to a close by summarizing what has been gleaned, checking this with participants. It reinforces the importance of what they have just given of themselves, for they have given of themselves, which is more than just their time. Participants now have the opportunity for refining their input and for helping to establish a consensus within this particular group. There is the question of what to do with the data generated. Tape transcription is usually completed as soon as possible after the session, and the moderator's notes will help to fill in any paralinguistic gaps. The researcher will manipulate and interpret this raw data. Each step in the process offers itself for scholarly discussion, drawing on the literature on focus groups.

Survey

Survey research enables a wide range of participants for a research project to be accessed. A sample, the size of which you will determine according to the requirements of your research and your ability to manage the numbers involved, is a given questionnaire on which they may record their responses to a number of questions that you have formulated. It is wise to avoid, or at least curtail, the possibilities of *yes* and *no* answers, but sometimes you do need some plain facts as well as subjective responses to issues. Surveys may be written, oral, social media-based (Facebook and so on) and electronic programs may be most helpful in getting your survey out to large populations of respondents (see, for example, Survey Monkey).

There are practical considerations to be addressed. If you do a mail survey, how will you get the addresses of the people you want to respond, and how can you ensure that they will respond to your request? A return-paid envelop may help, but this does not ensure its use. If you do a telephone survey, how will you get the telephone numbers, and how will you stop people hanging up on you before you even get to the survey bit, especially if they are already feeling badly done by as call centers may have been ringing them at most inconvenient times? Another complicating factor is how to record answers given over the telephone, especially if the questions are designed to be open ended. If you are using social media, how can you restrict your respondents to those people to whom your research is most relevant? Are the social media people that you intend to work with really the respondents that you want? If you are doing an electronic survey, how can you get the e-mail addresses of the people you want to contact, and how can you ensure that they will respond?

Once you have addressed such problems, you will give consideration to how you will collate the data that you have. The written responses have different characteristics from those of oral responses, electronic responses will have taken on the characteristic brevity of the tweet and the post, and electronic survey tools will have enabled you to have made some firm decisions about what you would have anticipated from respondents before you sent the survey out.

You may try what is somewhat derisively referred to as *the scatter gun* approach, working with what you actually manage to hit with your survey, but this may not help with the case that you will make for the trustworthiness of your research unless you can argue it convincingly for the examiner(s). You may use the *snowball* approach, where participants suggest other possible participants. You may use purposive sampling, where a particular group is specifically identified and approached by you (in person, by letter, by telephone, by social media, by electronic survey tools, or even something as simple as a notice on a cafeteria, common room, and staff room notice board).

Again, scholarly considerations are to be addressed, including the possible influences of the medium being used to gather the data. It is advisable to do a practice run of the survey before you do the final one so that you can see what, if any, problems emerge, and address them before you embark on your final one.

Observation

When used as a research technique, observation is more than just looking at things, or people, or things that people do. It means a certain selectivity, for not everything, or everyone, or everything that everyone does, can be encompassed in a single research project. By the same token, in qualitative research, observation technique is not to be restrictive, for it is designed to generate those rich descriptions so often referred to in research writing, rich because of the careful observations and detailed notes upon which they are based. On the one hand, observation technique is restricted to what can be observed and what volume of data may be managed; on the other, observation technique is open to unanticipated dimensions of what is observed and to their detailed and carefully noted characteristics. It is a decision that the observer makes on the basis of their understanding of the research substance, methodology, method, and technique adopted in the case concerned.

There are practical considerations of how the researcher will not be obtrusive in relation to what is being observed, and in such ways interfering with the very things being studied. At the same time, there are scholarly concerns of what is the observer effect, where the very presence of the observer in some may influence who or what is or are being observed. This then raises ethics considerations, for under no circumstances are specific people to be observed for research purposes without their knowledge and consent. The observer effect as a measure of trustworthiness of the research, then, presents a number of considerations to receive your scholarly attention, and your explanations of how they are to be addressed. Neither are you as a qualitative researcher working in a legal or moral vacuum, for if illegal or even unsociable behavior where any of the people being observed may be harmed in some way is observed, you are obliged to intervene. This may wreck your observation as research technique altogether, but this is an inescapable characteristic of the technique.

That does not mean that you cannot work with the data that you have up to that point, or use the fact that you had to call off the observation at that point, and then work with what you have at hand.

Field notes

The apparently simple technique of the researcher, be they ethnographers, observers, interviewers, or surveyors, making notes as they work in their research sites, is another of those more complex phenomena of research. Wolfinger's (2002) research on the making of field notes shows that, "...irrespective of any formal strategies for note-taking, researchers' tacit knowledge and expectations often play a major role in determining which observations are worthy of annotation" (p. 85). Etic and emic considerations come into play here, and the notion of the qualitative researcher not working in a vacuum is once again highlighted. You may use field notes as a technique on its own, or as a supplementary technique to others being used, but you will give scholarly considerations to the implications of your own understandings and research positioning when you introduce the field notes to your writing up of your research.

Wording or phrasing of documents

You will not attempt to deal with every document on the issue or issues that you are investigating, but will be selective in relation to topic, emphases, sources, and so on. You will end up reading more documents than you will use in your research, for some will come to the fore as being of more significance than others. Some will have already have their own prominence; others will have been the subject of scholarly inattention and your focus on them will help to refocus enquiry to enable other dimensions of what is under study to emerge for scrutiny.

At the most simple level, you may use the *Find* function of your word processing program to search for key words and the number in which they appear in a document. You may find, though, that the complexity of your data will require you to have a license or a copy of your own of software for this sort of qualitative research (see, for example, NVivo, in QSR, 2013). As you do this, you will be making decisions about what you will emphasize, and what you will pay little and least attention, ensuring that you make scholarly arguments for the decisions that you make.

Diaries/journals

Items in diaries or journals will give you the raw data for your research. You will not use the diaries or journals as complete entities for research purposes, but will identify specific items for your research. You may also simply use the *Find* function, as well as the relevant software in doing this. Again, the decisions that you make will be informed by your positioning of yourself as a researcher, and you will explain your reasoning as you proceed.

Photographs/film

You will select particular photographs and films, as well as particular details within those photographs and films as your data, explaining your reasons for your selection of these. You will be relying a good deal on your own understandings of the concerns of your research as you do this, and there is not a great deal in the way of software to help you in this. Researchers wanting to use software to help them in this find that the material, such as low resolutions and lack of clarity in the picture or film, itself presents some problems. This is the subject of current technological development, and it is worthwhile keeping abreast of this in the proceedings of conferences on such developments.

An annotated example

States the two techniques used at the outset

Moves straight into scholarly considerations of the problematic re the techniques

The written public record the documents provide has served to supply a rich resource of material for analysis, but I established a number of interviews and interview procedures as well. In doing so, I have drawn on the work of a number of scholars in the field, including Scheurich (1997), who points out that it is only from a positivist perspective that the research interview can be seen as an unproblematic method for gathering qualitative data (p. 61). I have not treated the analyses of the transcripts of taped interviews as verbatim, accurate representations of issues under discussion, but acknowledge that they are the result of what Scheurich (1997) describes as 'a creative interaction between the conscious/unconscious researcher and the decontextualised data which is assumed to represent reality or, at least, reality as interpreted by the interviewee' (p. 63). I have taken the opportunities that taped interviews and transcripts provide for multiple listening and focus and refocus on key points that called themselves to attention at later dates, a point raised by Thompson (1996, p. 7). I have been able to note disorders of discourse within and across government and whole [organisation] and [section] policies in my analysis, but I have not able to ascertain the extent to which each interviewee was able to let me see all. ...In posing the interview questions, I anticipated the role of the interviewee as providing responses which 'open up a horizon of possible meanings to be pursued during later analysis' (Kvale, 1996, p. 184). I have not tried to represent transcripts to be '... Taken as the embodiment of truth as an indisputable record of the interview' (Poland, 1995, p. 291), for I have not in this thesis set out to establish such a thing.

Discussion of data re reality and perceptions of reality

Notes considerations of how much an interview can tell a researcher

Explains limitations of the technique

All claims made supported by scholarly literature

It is the language in which the recall of these practitioners is couched that has been my focus, not the facts, perceived or otherwise, of their experience. This has allowed me to analyse the interviews according to sets of constructs based on themes and topics that emerges from the document analysis set against those of the interviews themselves. I have not questioned the veracity or otherwise of interviewee or document statements, but have considered them as discourses which constitute and are constituent of the discursive field in which participants operate. ... This process has allowed me to identify gaps between the written descriptions of practice and the action forms of organisational procedures and protocols as I matched them and set them side by side. I have used the techniques of analysis of public statements from a variety of organisational sites and interview transcripts primarily to generate as full a picture as possible of the practice of the organisation, generating descriptions of smaller networks within larger organisational ones. In doing so, I have been able to examine the implementation of national policy statements within an organisational context, as stated in my principal and subsidiary research questions.

Situates technique within own research methodology

Addresses limitations re relevance to own research

No reference to triangulation as this does not apply in this research

Signposting. Finishes on reference to research questions

References and citations given in the style required by that university.

The annotated example as a model

The candidate has given careful consideration to the problem aspects of techniques used, not taking them as simple or straightforward things to undertake. Methodological and practical considerations are taken into account, and done so in accordance with the methodology and method employed (there is no discussion of triangulation, for example, as this does not apply here).

The words used

- For the techniques themselves, the words that you will use are *I have used interviews/focus group/observation*, (and so on) *as tools to enable me to generate data...*
- Words like *method, approach*, and *methodology* are not to be used in relation to *interview/ focus group/survey* (and so on). If you do not keep the idea of techniques being separate from them, you will tend to conflate them and use them interchangeably, which really will not work.
- When you discuss technique, you will refer to the literature on the particular technique under discussion. Use expressions like: *drawing on the work of Thompson (1996) and Wolfinger (2002) I have....*

Suggested reading

Dianne Thompson's (1996) *The tape recorder as a mediating factor in research* is a detailed consideration of the less than neutral role of the recording device used in the research interview.

There is not a lot of new material on the conduct of focus groups in qualitative research, but Bloor, Frankland, Thomas, and Robson's (2001) *Focus groups in social research* gives a good overview.

This one is related to quality health care, but it really does examine some of the key features in quality survey research: Kelley, K., Clark, B., Brown, V., & Sitzia, J. (2003). *Good practice in the conduct and reporting of survey research.*

The best of the literature on observation is to be found in general research methods handbooks and guides, so explore these to inform your discussions on use of observation technique.

Nicholas Wolfinger's (2002). *On writing fieldnotes: Collection strategies and background expectancies* takes up a number of most salient points in relation to field notes, particularly for the person using ethnography method.

The *International Journal on Document Analysis and Recognition (IJDAR)* (Doermann, Kise, & Marinai, 2013) is dedicated to articles on processes, procedures, and developing software programs and document analysis. It provides timely scholarly contributions, as it says, "...Dealing with computer recognition of characters, symbols, text, lines, graphics, images, handwriting, and signatures."

Conclusion

Having reached this milestone of having the research technique identified, discussed, and planned for putting to use is significant progress. If you are going to implement some form of triangulation, you will use more than one technique in the generation of your data. It is from this point that you can embark on the next but most important practical step of the research: collecting the data. We will address this in the next chapter.

Hot Tip 7

As you search the literature for scholarly articles on the technique(s) you have opted to use, you will find gaps that, while perhaps annoying for you at this stage of your research progress, you will be able to fill with scholarly and professional journal articles and conference presentations of your own. Thompson's article on the recording device and the interview is one of the most recommended and cited articles on the topic, and it emerged as part of her own PhD studies. You could do the same.

Milestone 8: Collecting the data

8

Getting to data collection

One of the most appealing aspects of doing research is getting into the data collection stage, setting up interviews and interview questions, distributing surveys, tracking down and gathering documents in one place, doing transcripts, and so on. This is understandable, but some caution needs to be exercised in this regard. You will not complete all the reading and writing associated with the "Milestone 3: Getting Ethics Clearance" to "Milestone 7: Technique" chapters before you get into this chapter, but we recommend that you ensure that you have a thorough understanding at least of the methodology that you are using before you get to gathering the data. We have found that candidates who collect their data before they have a handle on the methodology then find that they have not collected the data that they have needed. Worse still, these candidates are then in some difficulty in data collected being analyzed in relation to the methodology with which they are to analyze this data. Remember, while it is useful to tease out the various elements of what constitutes your PhD for detailed discussion, all of them overlap and interweave.

Data collection and methodology

If you are to analyze your data in relation to phenomenology, for example, and you have not built in means by which to get data on the life worlds of your participants, you will be in a bind. The concept of lifeworlds is integral to phenomenology and data analysis. If you are basing your research on poststructuralism, you will be able to engage a knowledgeable discussion on the relationship between power and knowledge, discourses, subjectivities, silences, apparatuses of power, and so on. Given this, you will design your data collection around these things. Symbolic interactionism will take you into the world of objects, happenings, behaviors, and so on in people's lives, and the meanings they ascribe to such things. You will be focusing on constructivism in relation to ways meanings are constructed in the social world. Your supervisor will guide you in relation to the various features of your PhD activities to take this into account, and may urge delaying data collection until you have indicated to them that you have a good grasp of the methodology. It is worth taking their advice on this.

Data collection and method

Even so, you will now have a well-developed understanding of the method you are using. If you are using case study method, you will know that you will be working with a number of features that pertain to this case, and your data collection will include each of these. You will not rely on only one source of data, for a case study presumes more than one source. If you have opted for some sort of triangulation, you will need to have your strategies for this in place: what are the techniques that you intend to use for this purpose? There are many things to consider in relation to data collection when designing a case for research using this method.

If you are examining a discursive field, you will map the field in relation to a power–knowledge nexus, discourses that construct subjectivities, foregrounded and backgrounded discourses, the silences that apply, the apparatuses of power, the authority of those permitted to make statements on subjects, and so on. You need to have such considerations in place before you start collecting data.

If you are doing an ethnographic study, you will have made decisions in relation to your own positioning within the social group under study. You might live with the group, or visit at regular or irregular intervals. Whatever you decide, you will need a number of sources of data for analysis if you are to get as complete an ethnographic understanding as you can manage.

The techniques themselves are not necessarily particular to method; any number of methods may use the same techniques. Interviews are used in case studies, at the same time as they are used in discourse analysis, at the same time as they are used in ethnography, at the same time as they are used in narrative enquiry, and so on. The same applies to document analysis and other techniques: they may be used in any number of methodologies and methods. The point is that it is not the techniques themselves that are at issue in data collection, it is the ways in which they are used, particularly if they are used in conjunction with others.

Let us imagine for a moment that you are investigating a particular organization. Such a piece of research is open to a number of methodologies or methods being selected. To ensure that you are able to represent as complete a picture as possible of what you are researching, you will have made a number of decisions about the data collection techniques that you will use as appropriate to the decisions that you have made regarding methodology and method.

Given the nature of case study, you need to have a number of sources of data, and not just interviews with a given number of heads of a given number of sections in the organization, for example. Given the nature of discourse analysis, you will map the features of a discursive field in which the organization is situated. Given the nature of an ethnographic study, you will give representation of a wider number of cultural and social features that apply in relation to this group of people within an organization. A narrative enquiry implies the various and interconnected elements of stories of a number of elements with the organization, and so on. The point to be made is that whatever method you are working with, you will be concerning yourself with collecting data from a number of sources, even if you are doing this only from the perspective of triangulation.

Data collection and techniques

Regardless of methodology and method, in generating data from a number of sources for your research into this particular organization, you will look to the possibilities of a number of data collection techniques:

- You will perhaps also conduct interviews with underlings of the section heads you have interviewed.
- Perhaps you will also conduct interviews with users of what is produced or provided in those sections. Will you organize access to documents produced in relation to those sections... annual reports, Web pages, social media postings, advertisements, or promotions?
- You might want to look at formal and informal documents, such as copies of letters or e-mails or tweets from within or about those sections.
- Maybe diaries and journals present themselves as the sorts of data sources that you need. Can you get ethics-approved access to these?
- Will you want to survey as well as interview the people concerned in your research? If you do, will the survey be paper based, audio based, electronically based, or something else?
- Will you rely on photographic representations and films of activities of the section heads or will you want other personnel to be photographed and filmed as well?
- Will you videotape or audiotape the section heads, their underlings, and the products and services they offer being used?
- Will you supplement interviews, photographic and film material, documents, and correspondence with observations recorded in field notes?
- Would field notes serve as your primary data source, supplemented with photographs? Would these two be enough?
- Perhaps the content of your own research journal in which you record significant occurrences, thoughts, and perceptions about your research as you proceed from the outset to the end fits the bill as a data source.
- When you consider etic and emic aspects of your positioning within the research project, you become part of the data collecting exercise yourself. Are you part of the organization under study perhaps, or are you a complete outsider? Consider, you will ask different questions and get different data given insider knowledge and shared understandings with the people within the organization from the questions and data you will get as a stranger to the organization.

These sorts of considerations need to have been worked out before you start. Not only that, but you will tell your examiners about each of those that you take up, and how it relates to your collection of data for this research.

Data collection instruments

Whatever data collecting techniques you are using, the actual items associated with each is a data collection instrument. If you are using interview technique, the interview itself is the instrument. So too is the survey itself, the questionnaire, the audio or videotape, and so on. To make sure that you have an effective instrument to collect the data that you want, it is advisable to do a test run with a trial group before you use it with participants. In this way, you will be able to deal with any unforeseen issues with the instrument as these show up with the trial group.

An annotated example

The annotated example given below illustrates ways in which a candidate has taken up some of the issues involved in their discussion of issues related to data collection.

[Starts with topic sentence, establishing content of the section]

Van Manen (1990) states that in research processes, the avenue for gaining information or data may be varied, but leads to illuminating the phenomenon [under examination]. This gathering of data can take a diversity of forms, such as from those who have experienced it, from observations, from anecdotes, or from a number of other sources. Examples of these sources, given by van Manen (1990), are the use of art, diaries, journals or literature. No matter the avenue for the gaining of information, the outcomes lead to making visible perspectives on the nature of the phenomenon being studied (van Manen, 1990). … As I have chosen case study method, this has left me open, as a researcher, to using various methods of data collection (Hamel, Dufour S., & Fortin, 1993) through which I have constructed and then analysed the case. The use of open-ended surveys, focus groups and my own professional journal reflections as the tools for data collection culminate in the text being presented as a case study …

[Canvasses a number of possibilities for data collection]

[Moves into discussion of own data collection]

[Specifies questionnaire. Limitations of these]

Questionnaires: Questionnaires conducted have formed the basis of preliminary data gathering for analysis in my study. Participants' responses to questions have provided one source of data in my research. Reading and re-reading these questionnaire responses, I identified common themes and patterns of language indicating a range of issues faced during the early phase of participant experience. The challenge in focusing on this data was that the texts in the questionnaires did not provide enough depth to get to the heart of the story of participants' experience.

Given the nature of data that may be collected via questionnaires, I have sought to achieve a deeper understanding by incorporating a different form of data collection to gain a greater depth to that data. I considered that focus group discussions would enable this. I used the themes and patterns identified in the questionnaire data collected to develop questions for the focus groups. Silverman (2001) states that focus groups can rapidly provide data, more than observation can, while Flick (2002) stresses the 'interactive' nature (p. 120) of this form of data collection. Focus groups expanded the data collection and also provided rapid collection of data creating an interaction between this and the data from the questionnaires. Four focus groups were facilitated in this phase of data collection.

[Focus groups as another form]

[Benefits of focus groups supported by literature on research]

… A letter of invitation was sent inviting participation in one of the focus groups. There was a total of thirty-five participants, eight in Focus Group One, ten in Focus Group Two, ten in Focus Group Three and seven in Focus Group Four. Each participant was invited to attend one focus group session lasting approximately one and a half hours. The same facilitator was used for the four focus groups in order to maintain a measure of consistency in the way in which the groups were managed. The decision to use an outside facilitator was made for ethics reasons, which I have discussed in a following section. I briefed this facilitator prior to each session and

[Explains to the examiner how this was done]

provided him with a list of open-ended question. These questions were reflective of the themes which had emerged from my reading and re-reading of questionnaire data, and the synthesis that I had made of the overviews of the data collected from these questionnaires. While the facilitator pursued these themes with each focus group, he also allowed the group to elaborate or diverge from the questions he had before him if the topics were related to the focus of the transition experience and the challenges participants face during this phase. The focus groups were recorded on audiotapes and these were transcribed as outlined below. The use of a tape recorder rather than notes taken by the facilitator enabled an enhanced depth to the data, as suggested by Thompson (1996). The use of tape recordings also allow for revisiting the content and can provide details of utterances and allow the researcher the opportunity to improve transcripts by re-playing the tapes (Silverman, 2001).

Details of focus groups procedures

Reference to classic work on tape recorder

Journals as Data: Journals may be seen as material culture, which also includes letters and other personal communications, that form part of the resources from which data may be extracted in research (Silverman, 2001). He further points out that these documents can provide a rich source of data and are considered as a valuable record in the collection of qualitative research data. As part of my professional practice, I have maintained a professional journal. Each of these journals forms part of the data which I have included in my research. The data in my professional journals come from my personal observations over a period of seven years of working in the environment in which my research is situated. The content of these documents provide a form of field notes which became helpful to me as a researcher in formulating ideas and, as (Bryman, 2009) suggests, developing 'hunches' (p. 77) about the case under study. The journals include a range of texts which include my own observations about [the culture of the organisation] as well as informal interactions between myself and others within it.

Positioning self and journals as part of data collection

I took advantage of this 'naturally occurring' data (Silverman, 2001, p. 286,) and have incorporated relevant entries from this source as data in my study, where I have viewed that these add to the exploration and elucidation of the experiences of participants. In using of this data from my journals I take into consideration Silverman's (2001) words of caution that such naturally occurring data which I gained from situating myself in the field and observing and interacting with students can be influenced by my own views and that of the participants I have observed. I use these extracts from my journals as supporting data or data which relate to the themes which I have already established from the depth of data occurring in both the questionnaires and the transcripts from the focus groups. I discuss the strategies for the analysis of the data sources I have described here being the questionnaire data, focus group transcripts and data and my journals as documents in the following section.

Etic and emic considerations

Finishing on the topic of data collection from a variety of sources

Signposting

Citations given in the style required by that university.

The annotated example as a model

Not only does this example show ways in which the candidate has addressed issues of techniques for data collection, it also shows that they have maintained a position of a scholarly discussion of these, making no claims that are not supported by the literature on research. What is more, they have applied *The Fairy Tale Principle* here, with a clear topic sentence on data collection at the beginning of the section, explanation and development of the various dimensions of data collection in the following sentences, and a final reference to a depth of data emerging from the use of a variety of data sources. Another noteworthy feature of this example is its signposting at the very end, informing the examiner(s) of what is about to come (see also "Milestone 2: The confirmation or defence of candidature" chapter).

The words used

The words used here are of the most straightforward kind. There is no engagement with big philosophical, methodological, or method questions. This has already been done, and this milestone builds on the understanding that the answers to such questions have been dealt with. Much of what is written now is of a practical nature, telling the examiner the details of processes and procedures.

Suggested reading

The works suggested in the annotated example are most relevant to this aspect of writing your thesis:

Hamel, Dufor, and Fortin's (1993) *Case study method* has a detailed discussion of case study method, but it makes a number of pertinent comments on techniques, data collection, and data analysis as well.

Bryman's (2009) *Social research methods*, given its general discussion of the social research field, takes up issues of both data collection and analysis in your research area.

Both Silverman and Flick, who come up again and again as good resources, are worth consulting on this as well.

Conclusion

When you reach this chapter, you are reaching what we might call the business end of the PhD undertaking, and your language becomes more businesslike as well. You focus on details of the conduct of the research itself, but you maintain your scholarly stance of basing all that you say in the literature that you have been consulting since you started. The rest of the business end takes you into things like transcripts, identifying patterns that emerge from your studying of the data from their various sources, and making scholarly comment on them in light of the methodology that has informed you every step of the way up to this point.

Hot Tip 8

When you get to collecting data, make sure that your equipment works if you are recording in some way. Check that it is working before you go to wherever the recording is to take place, and if any of it is battery based, take along at least one set of spares. This applies to any of the parts that are to be used...lamps, cords, double adaptor electric plugs, film. Modern digital recording devices tend to take a lot of the guesswork out of successful recording, but Murphy's Law still applies: *If anything can go wrong, it will.* You may not get a second chance at interview, and it also tends to show you in a bad light as a researcher if the equipment doesn't work.

Milestone 9: Analyzing the data

9

Getting to data analysis

Having collected your data, you will make a start on analyzing it. Data analysis, for the qualitative researcher, means investigating data in a manner that enables researchers to perceive patterns, identify themes, find relationships between various phenomena or ideas, develop explanations, and interpret all of this in light of the theory that has been drawn upon in the conduct of the research.

There is a number of things that you will do in organizing this part of your PhD, and you will tell your examiners all about it. Now that you have reached this milestone, you are getting close to finishing. You will probably still be reading around the other milestones, with a view to finessing what you have so far so that you can finalize those chapters, but you will have broken the back of the PhD. Your reading on theory will now be applied to the data itself. Until you have done this, you will only have data, and not the new knowledge that you set out to create.

Before you do this, though, you will explain how you have organized the data to enable you to analyze it. Some candidates use software programs to help them identify patterns of themes, words, concepts, actions, procedures, and so on, that appear in the data, and to show their regular or irregular dispersion throughout what has been collected:

> *Using NVivo, I have been able to identify themes and patterns which have emerged from the data, from which I was able to create a series of matrixes, one matrix for each of the techniques of data collection employed... This enabled me to identify the points at which the data from the individual and focus group interviews had provided a depth of themes. At this point I moved to a single matrix into which I placed all individual and focus group data to check for commonalities and differences in each set of data. At this time I moved back to the data from the documents and added data relevant to the themes and patterns as well as content from my own journal entries. This resulted in a representation of the web of experiences for me to analyse.*

Others will sort material under various headings on their computers, using simple devices like spread sheets to record ways in which patterns may be identified:

> *I have taken questionnaire responses and constructed a number of categories on the basis of three of van Manen's (1990) four existentials, those of lived space, lived time and lived other. I have not employed the theme of lived body for reasons discussed in Chapter 4. I have used the software program EXCEL to count responses and on the basis of these generated visual images in the form of pie charts and graphs for descriptive purposes.*

There are those who will use very low-tech devices. They use large sheets of paper, copies of transcripts and documents, and scissors and tape. They cut out material that indicates emerging themes and patterns from such copies to paste onto the sheets under various headings that pertain to the research. They then work from these large sheets posted on pin boards:

> *I pasted four large sheets of butcher's paper around the walls of my room, each of which had a heading suggested by my reading and rereading of the data that I had collected. As patterns and themes became evident, I wrote a heading that included such suggested themes on the pages. Sub-headings further suggested themselves to me as I highlighted, using differently coloured highlighting pens for the purpose, details from the letters that I had examined. Over the ten years of the correspondence examined, a number of issues of concern were mentioned over and over again, and I highlighted these and used them to create sub-headings on each page. Under each of these, I pasted the items from the letters themselves, grouping them to illustrate the writers' concerns on these issues.*

There is a certain idiosyncrasy in all of this, as candidates work through their own ways of organizing their data:

> *In order to identify common patterns of language and the relationships between these patterns, I recorded by hand the key quotes and phrases onto sheets of paper from which I was able to develop a picture of the social worlds described by participants. With further reading and re-reading of the texts I have been able to plot patterns and relationships between key issues that I have identified.*

The following explanation of a candidates' organizing their data leads them into the analysis itself as based on poststructuralist theory given by Foucault:

> *I had known from the outset that, having generated all this data, I would have to organise it in some way. Foucault's (1974) suggested 'grids of specification' (p. 49) in relation to his own analyses of where different kinds of discursive features—such as those of madness, the body, and so on—helped me with this. He suggests that with the use of such grids it is possible to discern where and how things are 'divided, contrasted, related, regrouped, classified, derived from one another ...' as objects of particular discourses. I adapted a use of grids as part of my own analyses of discourses, precisely because they facilitated the sorts of discernment Foucault suggests.*
>
> *I drew up twelve grids...to enable me to deal with large amounts of data in a systematic way. I had explored the possibilities of computer programs for such processes but did not use them for I felt it did not allow for the depth of analyses required in my research. I wanted conceptualisations associated with naming and positioning as normalising strategies, not just naming, to be the focus of this research. I felt that computer-generated systems of recurrent words and phrases, even if they were associated with specific time frames, a limitation on this work. Once the grids were in place, I could identify points at which naming and positioning strategies came into focus, such as that of the settling on the generally accepted terms in favour of possible others at any particular time, and where they disappeared, converged or*

diverged within discourses. I could identify silences at some points within discourses and points at which privileging of discourses would occur at others.... The grid based on globalisation, for example, called up conceptualisations of signs, logos and customers within discourses of developing capitalist practices, but the grid based on policy also called up conceptualisations of globalisation and salient aspects of it. The result for me was what (Foucault, 1973b) describes as a 'solid grid of kinships that define the general configuration of knowledge...' (p. 74). I constructed these grids as I read through the data, allowing headings to suggest themselves as issues, questions or themes recurred within the texts I was examining. Even so, the use of grids is not to be seen as an imposed structure on networks of discourse. The grid is a data organisational device I developed and used to facilitate my analyses, to help me to keep track of my explorations of the number of texts generated and discourses analysed in the course of this research, and to provide a number of points of reference within texts.

All such activities demonstrate orchestrated and systematic ways of dealing with data. Whatever you decide to do, detail your activities in the early part of this chapter so that the examiner knows exactly what you have done to organize the raw data for systematic analysis in accordance with the theory that you have drawn upon to inform your research.

Data analysis and methodology

Your methodology is the theoretical basis of your research. If you are using post-structuralism, you will analyze your data according to ways in which such things as discourses, discursive, fields, normalization, regimes of truth, power and knowledge relationships, silences, and so on, are made visible in the data that you have collected. If you are using phenomenology, you will analyze your data according to ways in which the lifeworlds of participants are evidenced, their lived experience in general and lived self, lived time, lived space, and lived other, in particular. Symbolic interactionism means that you will analyze your data in relation to the interpretation of significant symbols in the worlds of your research participants. The data that indicate their construction of social and cultural meaning are the words they use in the processes of interpretation they engage. You will analyze your data with a focus on individual responses to meaningful symbols derived from individuals' wider social world, with that wider social world backgrounding responsive interpretations under study.

An annotated example

The following is a heavily abridged reproduction of the candidate's theoretical discussion that leads in to their analysis of the data, but it serves to illustrate the way that they have engaged theory to deal with data.

Establishes what data analysis is

Immediately positions data analysis in relation to methodology of phenomenology

Scholarly discussion drawing on relevant literature

Inserts self to discussion

> I have focused on themes that have emerged from the data in relation to the lived time, lived space, lived other, and lived self of lived experience of [the participants in my research]. The lifeworld existential, lived time, is described by van Manen (1990) as subjective time rather than being measured by clock time in an objective sense. It is 'our temporal way of being in the world', according to van Manen (1990, p. 104), who also makes the point that it is through the body that lived time is experienced. Merleau-Ponty (1962) stresses the importance of this last point in relation to lived time, arguing that it is through the body that there is an experience of a past and a future, this being the basis of temporal experience of the world. Sartre (1956) states that to be intelligible, temporality requires 'the structure of selfness' (p. 195) and in this sense turning to phenomenology to study the past, present and future presents as a focus on the being itself. Taking this point into consideration, I have given consideration to temporality in relation to the being itself, and I have done this in the context of lived time of lived experience on which my research is focused.

Here, the candidate presents data that pertain to the concept of lived time in relation to participants in the research. They present similar theoretical discussions of phenomenology before going on to analyze the data in relation to lived space:

Teases out features of this aspect of the theory for focus

Discussion made relevant to this research

> A traditional notion of space relates to length and height or the distance between places (van Manen, 1990). Space, according to Heidegger (1962) is not considered 'to be found in the subject' (p. 146) but the subject itself 'is spatial' (p. 146), arguing that it is the experience of space and the encounter of space, and not the space of and by itself, which gives meaning and understanding to the lived experience. Lived space in the context of life world existentials is experienced as pre-verbal (van Manen, 1990), not being obvious to experience but coming into consciousness when reflecting on an experience. It is experience which is affected by the space in which a person exists (van Manen, 1990). Lived experience of lived space in the context of my research is reflected in the meanings which participants attach to the space in which they find themselves.

Again, what follows is data is extensively analyzed in relation to such theoretical concepts of lived other:

Establishes significance of this re own research

Continues to keep discussion relevant

> I have focused on lived other, the lifeworld existential suggested by van Manen (1990) which has as its focus the 'Lived relation we maintain with others in the interpersonal space that we share with them' (p. 104). … I have engaged the analysis of the data in light of this lifeworld existential as presenting another range of challenges in lived experience of XXX. In this chapter, I have discussed these experiences and the challenges which are faced by participants in my research in relation to lived other in lived experience, which, as Merleau-Ponty (1962) suggests, views people in the world as being linked through significant relationships. Given this, my analysis of [the data] has enabled me to provide insights which I have not found to be represented in the current literature

> in this field. The experience of other in the world is discussed by Sartre (1956) as ways in which human beings are revealed to themselves and to others, and it is through the lived relations with others that human identity is created. It is this idea of lived other, which is the focus of my analysis in this section of my thesis.

The theoretical discussion of lived self provides the basis for the end of data analysis in this thesis and follows the pattern already established:

> I have focused on the lifeworld existential that van Manen (1990) has identified as lived self. I have particularly focused on the emotional aspect of lived self ... in relation to corporeal and sensory associations as affecting both the mind and the body in human perception of the world; that the mind is located in the body and inextricably linked with it. In relation to my own research, lived self is reflective of physical, emotional and social changes which the participants view as part of their lived experience. Merleau-Ponty (1962) suggests that the body, while it may be considered as being made up of features such as muscle, skin, and bone, is also made up of an earthly or human aspect of living, and that this is intertwined with the mind. Lived body is considered by Merleau-Ponty (1962) as ways in which human beings are bodily in the world, as the world is interpreted through bodily, sensorimotor skills and intentionality. In my research the themes associated with lived self relate particularly to the sensory associations participants experience. The emotions particularly play a key role in participants' descriptions of their experience, and how they make sense of this as lived experience.

Maintains style, tone, and manner of data analysis

References and citations given in the style required by that university.

The final activity of the data analysis is informed by theory and at every step is tied to the methodology of phenomenology used in this research.

The annotated example as a model

The candidate has been most punctilious in ensuring that the very large amount of data used has been tied very closely to the methodology, leaving the examiner(s) in no doubt about how and why they have done this. They have integrated theory and data in the ways that research at PhD level demands, and they have never once lapsed in their focus on this.

The words used

- *I have focused on the...* (in reference to the themes identified for discussion)
- *I have focused on the* (in reference to the theory under discussion)
- *The data indicate...* (making it clear that claims made come from data and not opinion or belief)

- *Participants* (descriptions, experiences, writing, or whatever constitutes the data being used)
- *Transcripts of interviews indicate* (making it clear that there are no unsupported claims being made).

Suggested reading

Consult the works that you have used so far, both general texts on research in general, and specific texts on research in your field. There are others that may prove useful to you:

Grbich's (2013) *Qualitative data analysis* has stood the test of time, first published in 2006 and now in its second edition. It ties each part of the data analysis canvassed in with particular methodologies.

Bell's (1995) *Doing your research project* has a particularly helpful chapter called *Interpretation and presentation of the evidence.*

Others' theses will also have examples of what the candidates did, and how they wrote about it.

Conclusion

There is an almost irresistible temptation to dive joyfully into the data that you have collected and discover and point out patterns and themes that emerge in your reading of them. It is one of the most pleasant aspects of your research project. You would be seriously ill advised to make such a dive leaving your theoretical considerations behind. The two are inextricably linked, and your explicit linking of them in well informed discussion of theory is what is going to make your PhD a great success. Trying to present one without the other is not the way to go at all.

Hot Tip 9

Remember the people who have been good enough to volunteer to participate in your research, and show your respect for their doing this for you by making sure that you use what data they have provided for your research. This does not mean that you have to use every word of their interviews, surveys, questionnaires, letters, journals, dialog, or whatever, for that is just not possible. It does mean, though, that you ensure that you use at least some part of what they have so generously offered you.

Milestone 10: Drawing conclusions and making recommendations

10

Why draw conclusions and make recommendations?

It is when you reach this milestone that you deal with some of those *so what?* questions in relation to your PhD. It is not enough to show that you are able to design a research program at postgraduate research level and carry it out. You also need to be able to show that you can make logical arguments from what new knowledge you have generated. You also need to be able to show that you can see why and how the new knowledge you have generated contributes to your field's current store of it, and why this is significant. You have already dealt with issues of the significance of your research, probably in your first chapter, and this chapter will enable you to confirm your argument about that significance.

Getting to the conclusions and recommendations

You will make a case for your research having indeed been successful in achieving what it set out to do. This requires some summarizing and revisiting of what you have done. At this point, it is advisable to revisit your introductory chapter (if you have already written it; some of us leave it until we have reached this Milestone to write that chapter), to pull out the various points you have made about your research. You can then address them here as successfully completed. That way you will have in effect bookended the thesis: what you said at the beginning and what you are saying at the end will match.

Remembering that you started out with the idea of making your own contribution of some significance to an existing body of knowledge, as you summarize just how you have done this, you will acknowledge that what you have here is only a small part of completing the knowledge that currently exists in this field, as you have addressed that gap in the literature that you pointed out when you did the literature review. There will be other gaps, ones that have been beyond the scope of this one thesis, and you will point this out. It is possible, indeed highly probable, that as you have addressed the gap identified, you have raised further considerations that further research would be required to address. You will make recommendations about what it is that you have discovered for others to take up, perhaps in drawing on your work to inform theirs. As you do this, you will maintain your own scholarly stance and represent your conclusions and recommendations in the same language that you have used throughout the thesis.

Milestone Moments in Getting your PhD in Qualitative Research

An annotated example

In the following example, the candidate has taken up the idea of the limitations of their research and explored this in some detail in relation to the conclusions and recommendations made. Note that this candidate has chosen to use passive voice in their writing, as urged by their principal supervisor.

The researcher acknowledges that there are limitations to this research, which also suggests opportunities for future research. These limitations are briefly outlined below.

Firstly, while the cases in this research span a range of [cases] — based on demographics such as location, the number of employees, annual sales volume and industry classifications, ownership and so on — all are considered as eco-environmental friendly and are labelled as green firms by XXXX authorities. To some extent they form their own category as successful XXXX pioneers in [this country] and they do not represent or reflect the general business community in respect to going green and sustainable development. Future research endeavours would be advised to attempt to include a mixed population of firms and rules for classifying green firms to extend the transferability of the research results to other contexts or settings.

Secondly, this research is an attempt to develop a taxonomy of environment motivations, stakeholder identification and firms' green marketing frameworks using a qualitative, inductive method. While case study method is more than capable of exploring and developing a deeper understanding of the nuances suggested by the research questions, it does draw boundaries around knowledge claims and limits generalisation of the phenomenon under study to the wider industry scene in [this country]. One of the problems encountered in this research is that it has relied on self-narration of the interviewed managers, even though data from other sources were also used and verified. Future researchers would be advised to pursue a different triangulation of research methods (Jick, 1979) combining more [sources of data to supplement and illustrate the data generated here]. Such sources may be focus groups of employees across the firm and quantitative-based data such as surveys of important factors and Likert-type scales of those important factors influencing firms to go green [generated from] among employees, suppliers and customers across the value chain to provide a more robust basis for theory building.

Further, throughout the research it is assumed that the motivations of the interviewed general managers or founders of the firms are the prevailing motivations within the firm. In a typical collective culture, this assumption may be sound, but there is also evidence that economic progress is accompanied by a shift in values away from collectivism towards individualism (Hofstede, 1983). As pointed out by McGee (1998), there is the possibility of conflict between managers, as each functional manager can be subjected to pressure from different stakeholders and develop different motivations, which can bring coordination and control problems. This suggests that empirical studies that would measure the prevailing motivations within a firm, rather than the specific motivations of a particular manager such as the owners or founders or general managers

Left-margin annotations:

- Links limitation to recommendation
- Gives scholarly reason for recommending future research
- Scholarly discussion of case study method and the way it has been used in this research, referring back to method chapter and research questions
- Recommendations confirm candidate's grasp of possibilities for the conduct of trustworthy research
- Positions recommendations within wider research field

Right-margin annotations:

- Signposting, acknowledging limitations as bases for recommendations
- Specifies limitation in details
- Refers back to initial statements about the purpose of the research from the first chapter
- Scholarly reflection on own research
- Identifies further gaps that have emerged as the research has proceeded
- Supports position on the basis of what is in the literature
- Recommendation for further research based on issues of method, validity, and techniques

Annotation	Text	Annotation
Recommendations quite specific, not generalised	in this research, be conducted. This concern might be addressed by collecting and aggregating other managers' perceptions and opinions within each firm. Leaving this data collection technique aside, a clear outcome of this research is that the environmental attitudes, expectations and motivations of managers and, especially, of top managers, constitutes an important role for explaining the environmental proactivity and marketing orientation of a firm.	Finishes on re-statement of significance of this research
Reaffirms the significance of this research while acknowledging areas for future exploration in recommendations made	Despite the narrow focus and empirical work as outlined above, this research contributes significantly to understandings of ways in which firms perceive and deal with green marketing in relation to operational, environmental and marketing considerations in [this country]. The greening matrix proposed in this thesis is capable of accommodating explorations of the whole of firms' greening processes, with stakeholder identification, different motivation dimensions, possible greening approaches and marketing practices, and actors and factors influencing this. The credibility and generalisability of firms' greening processes in [this country] suggests itself as the subject of future research.	

References and citations given in the style required by that university.

The annotated example as a model

The candidate has been open and frank in their discussions of their work here. The stance is scholarly, based on the literature, and presenting an informed, balanced, and reflective account of what they have achieved in their research. They do not make claims of having solved all problems or addressed all issues that have emerged in relation to the phenomena under study. What is perhaps more important, they do not in any way suggest that they have conducted so complete and comprehensive a study as to suggest a definitive piece of research that closes the door on further work in the field. This is an important acknowledgment in relation to the sort of contribution to knowledge in this field that has been offered. At the same time, and rather importantly, they have struck just the right sort of authoritative tone to suggest that they have offered is acceptable in the first instance to the examiners, and then to the wider research community. The last paragraph alone would impress an examiner with its informed confidence in the work presented for them to assess.

The words used

- *I have laid out some prominent issues related to this reform as it has been implemented, with a discussion of research outcomes and issues still to be faced, which I have outlined below.*
- *In my selection of this as my research site I have limited my research to a particular group of participants…*
- *This feature of my research gives rise to the possibilities of further research in the form of a comparative study involving differently characterized participants involving different circumstances, such as …*

- *My research indicates that while policy statements and curriculum documents specify the skills to be developed in students, and the strategies to be employed by teachers, the ways in which they have been grounded in their profession means that much still needs to be done, as discussed below.*
- *An unexpected outcome of my research has been the inattention shown by those in authority to negative influences operating on participants concerned, and I recommend that such issues be highlighted and investigated further.*

Suggested reading

There is little in the literature on writing the conclusion chapters to theses apart from the more general books and handbooks on conducting research that you are already consulting, but there is one journal article that particularly stands out:

David Bunton's (2005) *The structure of PhD conclusion chapters.*

Conclusion

Reaching this milestone is a cause for serious celebration. There is still much for you to do, and it can be tedious and time-consuming as you prepare all that you have just written for printing and submission in accordance with the requirements of your university, but you have nailed it now, and deserve all the congratulations that you care to think of. It can be a difficult chapter to write, for there is a temptation to view what you have written in previous chapters as evidence of research conducted with rigor and vigor. This is not the case, for what is self evident as far as you are concerned is to be made explicit to the examiner(s). You are to make it clear that, while this is a significant piece of research, it is still a part, however large or small, of the bigger picture of research in the field, and that while it may be drawn on by other scholars, it is not by any means a definitive study of what has been researched by you and is being researched by others. This chapter requires you to maintain the same scholarly tone that you have used in all of the previous chapters, drawing on the literature to support any and all claims that you make, and being specific in conclusions and recommendations made.

Hot Tip 10

This is the last chapter that your examiner(s) will read, and it is your last chance to have them take their academic leave of you as impressed by the quality of your work. Make the most of this chance.

Milestone 11: Finishing, submitting, and examination

11

Having successfully reached every milestone, and having rightly congratulated yourself and celebrated getting to this point, there is more thing for you to do. One of the chapters that is still to be written is the first chapter, if you have left it till now. This is the one in which you set out how you got to the point of deciding upon the research, the significance of it, and so on. Many candidates write this chapter after the others have been written.

Bookending the thesis

When the first and last chapters are treated in this way, we can see it as a process of bookending the thesis, where the statements of the first chapter match those made in the final one. The first chapter establishes a number of bases for undertaking the research to begin with, and candidates who write this chapter at the beginning of their candidature find themselves in a largely speculative position, for they have not yet explored the details of their work in relation to the extensive literature they have consulted. If you have already written the chapter, though, this is the point at which to revisit it, to ensure that it conforms with the scholarly writing style and conventions of research writing that you have steadily developed as your writing of the thesis has proceeded. As with every other chapter in your thesis, all claims are to be based on evidence from the literature, with no assertions or speculations included. The task may be facilitated by setting up the headings and subheadings in your final chapter, and reproducing them as a structure for the first one. In this way, the possibilities for the research that you outline for the first chapter are matched with the conclusions from the research that you outline in the final chapter.

Completing the thesis and submitting

It is never too early during candidature to think about the end point. Too often we see candidates with a completed or near completed thesis not submitting at that time. Literature concerning the noncompletion and delay of submission of theses suggest that this is a complex area influenced by a variety of issues, including institutional and environmental factors, finance, the nature of the supervision, gender, race, and matters related to candidate characteristics, such as a tendency toward procrastination. Even when candidates have managed to navigate such issues there are some students who sit on a completed or near completed thesis. In Europe, this is referred to as ABS (All But Submitted) Syndrome. In North America, it is referred to as ABD (All But the Dissertation). Others refer to it as *the jelly wall.* If this applies to you, you need to identify what is stopping you from submitting. In our experience, the major factor here is the fear of being examined. We have candidates who have worked so hard and developed such in-depth knowledge that they suffer from "the more they know the less they think they know" and are convinced that an examiner will assess them as not being knowledgeable enough. Others are concerned that the findings were not what was expected and feel that the thesis is weak.

You are guaranteed to encounter both problems and opportunities when conducting your research which are peculiar to your undertakings and you will develop new ways of solving them. You will encounter peculiarities and idiosyncrasies of subjects that do not fit conventional moulds or stereotypes. It is useful to remind yourself that colleagues in the research community will want to know about this sort of thing, so that the new knowledge that you have generated is disseminated, and new knowledge developed that is built on yours. After all, you were never given all that support just to keep these new discoveries to yourself. If you have engaged the literature, conducted rigorous research, and developed a defensible argument, you will pass.

Viva voce

There are universities across a number of countries that require candidates to defend their research in an oral presentation, sometimes before the thesis is submitted for examination. This process is called Viva Voce. This is the point at which you present, discuss, and defend your research to a panel of research experts. You may expect questions from the panel that test your knowledge of the area under study, and about what you have researched, why you have researched it, how you have researched it, and ways in which you have addressed any problems that have emerged in the process. This may take an adversarial tone, or it may not, depending on the university and indeed the individual or collective panel members. The thing to remember is that the panel is trying to establish the depth of your knowledge and understanding of research processes, protocols, and conventions. It is not personal; it is a professional engagement with the wider research community. Remember that at this stage of your project, you are an expert in the field, in all probability more expert than some of the panel members, so relax into it and enjoy being taken so seriously by serious colleagues. As terrifying as this prospect may be to you right now, it is worthwhile to remember that they are not your enemy, and you are about to be admitted to equal status with them.

Conventions observed

You will have perhaps given your *Notice of Intention to Submit*, or some form of it, as required by your university, so you have a self-imposed deadline to meet as you come to the conclusion of your candidature. When you establish the date for submission, remember to include in your calculations the various demands on you at this point. There are certain conventions to be taken into account when you get to finalizing the thesis.

You will acknowledge the invaluable advice and assistance from your supervisors (and you will have already made sure that the scholarly work of your supervisor(s) has been consulted, cited, and referenced in this thesis of yours), naming them with their formal titles and starting with the principal supervisor. You might consider acknowledging the assistance you have received from librarians, research and graduate office people, fellow students, indeed all those who have freely given of their time even though they were not your supervisors. If you have interviewed, photographed, filmed, lived with, observed, or in any other way dealt with people who have provided you with your data, you will acknowledge any and all of them, for none of it would have happened without them. You will acknowledge the debts of gratitude that you have generated, given all the wonderful people who have been behind your endeavors along the way, such as all those supportive family members and friends. While these are standard conventions, there are no standard expressions for these...they come from you and what you feel. It is not part of the conventions to slight or insult anybody; far better to leave people with whom you have might have had issues along the way out of your considerations in your acknowledgment piece, or to be less than effusive in your acknowledgment of them.

And then there is the possibility of a dedication. This can only be determined by you, with the right words in which to express it.

Given the intensely personal nature of these features of your thesis, we have not given an annotated example. You may find that the ways in which others have done them useful as guides when you read them in their theses.

Editing and formatting

If only one of your supervisors is a good editor, then you are in luck. Even if you are a good proof reader yourself, it is always difficult, if not impossible, to proof read your own work successfully. You really need another pair of editorial eyes to read over your work. Not everybody has well-developed editorial skills, though, and if you can afford an editor, it is a good idea to use one. Some universities provide an allowance for their PhD candidates' use of professional editors, especially for those candidates whose first language is not that of the country in which the PhD is being undertaken.

You will need to check that your citations and references match. Even if you have been using good bibliographic software, it is possible that you have made an error or two when you have entered works used on the database, and this needs checking. Highlight the citations on your hard copy, and check each one against what is in the bibliography. It helps if you work with a partner.

If you have used Styles consistently throughout your writing, your Table of Contents will be done for you at the click of a key. If you have not, you have a laborious task ahead of you if you have to do it manually; best to go back into the document and redo headings and subheadings using the Styles function on your word-processing program so that the computer does your Table of Contents for you.

The university will have its own template and set of conventions for you to follow, such as a signed statement from you regarding the originality and ethical conduct of the research, a signed statement from your principal supervisor signing the thesis off as ready for examination (or not, if that is what they think and you are submitting it against their advice…it happens) formats for setting out required pages, especially at the beginning, attachments, and so on. They will also specify how the examinable document is to be printed and bound, and the number of copies they require from you. You will familiarize yourself with all of these and comply with requirements.

There is another function of word-processing programs, Auto-summarize, that we have found to be little used by research students, but it is extremely useful when you want to get an abstract for a larger piece of work. Given the size of your thesis, and the various dimensions of it, it may be difficult to frame the abstract in just the right words and within the word limit specified by your university. Auto-summarize will summarize the thesis according to what you specify—10%, 20%, 50%, 75%, or the number of words (250, 500, 1000), or whatever—so that you have something to work with even if it is not quite what you want. A number of our own students have done this with success.

After examination

The best part, of course, is when you get your examiners' reports back, and we would anticipate that this take no more than 3 months. Examiners are now asked to commit to this time frame before accepting a thesis for examination and generally adhere to it. This is when you really get to the final bit. It is not unusual for a thesis to come back from examiners as passed, with no changes to be made, but this does not always happen. It is also possible that a thesis comes back as not passed, but this is extremely rare. What is more likely is one of two other things.

It may come back with the examiners asking for a rewrite and resubmission. While this is not the best of all possible outcomes, it is not as bad as it might seem at first. The examiners will specify what they find in the thesis to be unsatisfactory, and it is only these things that you will have to address, working with your supervisors, before you resubmit for re-examination. This usually results in either a pass with certain more changes to be made (but only in relation to what they originally specified) to the satisfaction of the principal supervisor, or a panel convened in your faculty, department, or school. When this is done to their satisfaction, this is usually the end of the examination process in this eventuality.

It may come back with a pass, on condition that specified requested changes are made to the satisfaction of the principal supervisor, or a panel convened in your faculty, department, or school. When this is done to their satisfaction, this is usually the end of the examination process in this case.

Having satisfied the requirements of the examiners, and your faculty, school, or department, you will have the required numbers of your thesis bound according to requirements (and yours, if you want extra ones for your own purposes), and submit the final copy electronically to your country's digital theses program. This is where all theses are stored electronically and accessed electronically by other scholars or interested people.

You will then apply for inclusion in a graduation ceremony at your university. In many cases, you cannot officially use your new title until after graduation. This does not mean that you have to participate in the ceremony itself. You can have the degree conferred in your absence. Then you are finished.

Suggested reading

The best reading to inform the writing of acknowledgments and dedications is what has been written by others, so have a look at what they have written to inspire and guide your own. You can do this via the digital theses program, or go to the hard copies kept in your library or research and graduate studies office. If you are experiencing what some refer to as the jelly wall, the following may be of some help:

Baker, J. (1998) gives some consideration to this as it appears in candidates in the US.
Latona, K., and Browne, M. (2001) consider candidate reluctance to submit completed theses in Australia.
Park, C. (2005) looks at the situation in the UK.

Conclusion

Once you have written the thesis itself, there is still some work to be done before you can submit. It is wise to allow yourself plenty of time to meet the deadline that you impose upon yourself when you give your university your *Notice of Intention to Submit* or its equivalent at your university. Allow for final proof reading, editing, checking of citations and references, signing of required documents, writing of those important bits of the acknowledgment and the dedication, and allow time for printing and binding. Even after thesis submission, there may be a 3-month wait for its return, and some more time may need to be allowed for so that you can meet examiners' specified requirements. After that, it may be a month or more before your university holds one of its graduation ceremonies, where your degree will be conferred and after which you may officially use your new title. That's a great day!

Hot Tip 11

That thesis of yours will be a public document after it has been examined—and those words that you use in the acknowledgments and dedication will assume a greater importance than you might think when you first write them at submission stage—so take a long-term view of the implications of these very telling words of yours.

Milestone 12: Publishing out of your thesis

12

Purpose of publishing

While the focus of research efforts is on getting the research done and the thesis written, there is an extra dimension of activities to be considered in the process of undertaking a higher degree by research. This is getting yourself published, for it is important in positioning yourself as a published researcher, aware of the academic conventions associated with what it means to be a researcher. Your degree is, after all, part of some sort of national research training scheme, primarily government funded to provide university places such as yours to build your country's research capacities. This means that you develop doctorly habits and stances, engaging doctorly activities and attitudes to such activities. To engage this dimension of your work, you set yourself up with several published journal articles prior to submitting your thesis which will then position you ahead of the pack when starting to apply for academic positions. There will be postdoctoral positions for which you might apply, as well as the possibilities of a more senior rather than junior academic positions becoming more achievable when you have not only your degree and its title but also a publications list to back your application(s).

Given this, it is worth giving some consideration to the purposes of publishing your work. First, it is to contribute to the field of knowledge in your academic area. This allows you to meet your obligations, as a person in the privileged position of being a researcher in your field, of making public your contribution to the generation of knowledge. Your place is not funded to allow you to indulge yourself in the immensely satisfying pursuit of knowledge for you alone. You are obliged to disseminate the outcomes of your work. There is a personal dimension as well, though, for your publications list enables you to enhance your own position as a researcher as you put your work out to a wider audience than the one provided by the examiners of your thesis.

Publication type

You may reach that wider audience in a number of ways: a scholarly journal article; a chapter of an edited scholarly book; a refereed academic journal article; a professional journal article; a newspaper or a magazine article; a scholarly book. These may be part of electronic means of dissemination as well, particularly as so many journals now make their articles available online, and publishers are exploiting the possibilities of e-books. There are also other possibilities: you can disseminate the outcomes of your work in specifically designated and designed Web pages; and you can blog, Twitter,

Instagram, and Facebook. So mainstream are these last that they have even become new verbs in the language. You might consider designing a board game for budding researchers, or create an app for modern phones, tablets, and iPads.

In developing your publications list, the most usual path is a traditional one that begins with a scholarly journal article, followed by a chapter of book, and then a book. You may also decide that part of your job is to contribute to professional debates and discussions in your field, and publish a professional journal article, one that will be accessed by practitioners. This sort of article will not be received as top drawer publications by the powers that be in academia, but it is important in establishing yourself as an authority in the field that academia is meant to service. An extension of this, of course, is a newspaper or magazine article. The ultimate aim, though, is to attract the attention of publishers who would be prepared to publish your work in the form of a scholarly book. Your publications list is evidence for them that you can do this, and that they can take a punt on you.

We are talking about scholarly work here, so it is worthwhile revisiting the definition of research as generating new knowledge or using existing knowledge in new ways (which means generating new knowledge in any case). You are the one doing this, and nobody else is studying what you are from your perspective. If this were not the case, you would not have been offered your PhD candidature. Remember, nobody else has your knowledge, and everybody else in your field wants to know what you know.

Even so, your candidature has two components: the research itself and the thesis that presents that research. The thesis is a document presented for examination, written for the examiners only. It is not for the wider academic public, even if it is placed on your university's library shelves and electronically deposited in a national digital theses program. It is not for your supervisor(s). It also has a particular tone and phrasings that are consistent with the requirements of this document. It has an examinee's tone, and voice and phrasings, because the thesis is written according to conventions of the research thesis genre. It is a quite distinctive and particular form of text type that does not exist anywhere else. Even so, it has subgenres within that genre; each chapter has its particular function and fits within a particular sort of construction: situating the study, literature review, methodology, method and techniques, data analysis, conclusions and recommendations for further research. This sort of configuration belongs in no other genre, although certain bits may apply in things like essays or research reports.

Genre

It is this concept of genre that is the key to publishing out of your thesis. The central features of genre need to be kept in focus. Genres are text types with established conventional forms and characteristics that are instantly recognizable to all writers and readers of them. Each genre is informed by its own sense of purpose and sense of audience, which determines not only the content but also the tone and voice of the writing.

A common misconception is that the genres in scholarly writing are the same, and that distinctions in genres can be blurred. This gives rise to another misconception, and that is that the audiences for theses and scholarly articles, scholarly books and chapters, and scholarly publications in electronic media, and so on are also the same. They are not.

When it comes to publishing work out of a thesis, a most common mistake is the failure or inability to distinguish between the genre of the thesis and the genre of the research article, or book, or book chapter, and so on. The writer who does not make the distinction tends to take what is in the thesis and submit a shortened version of it for publication, without genre considerations. That writer leaves in all the methodology, all the method, and all the techniques and strategies material. They also leave in all the information for examiners, retaining the examinee's tone and voice, and in doing so neglect the needs of the new and different audience, ignoring the advice from the editors of the journals and the book publishers.

There is a certain irony in all of this. One of the difficulties in writing a thesis is that of unlearning the genre of the book or the research article when we are so immersed in these. We see how they are written, and just as we were taught when we were still in school, we pick up on them as models for our own research writing. Then we have to ditch them as we learn the genre of the thesis that is to be written and submitted for the purposes of the PhD. We have to write every word as addressing the research question(s) at the same time as we write every word as addressing the examiner(s). We have to learn to write the literature review as positioning our research for the edification of examiners, not as a list of everything that we have read. Then when we come to write our own scholarly articles, we have to discard the genre of the thesis and turn again to the genre of the article or the book chapter, book, and so on.

The point to be emphasized is that the genres of the thesis and other forms of scholarly writing are different from each other. The scholarly book or chapter of edited scholarly books is constructed around chapters with content based on and organized around themes, issues, and arguments. These chapters may be organized along linear or stand-alone features, as in a scholarly book, edited book, or a chapter of book. Unlike the thesis, the purpose is not for examination, the audience is not the examiner(s), and the tone and voice are not those of an examinee.

Working with the concept of genre, though, opens up a whole new field of publishing possibilities. Not the least of these is specific content for consideration. There is what your research is telling you, so that is one of your first considerations. You might perhaps consider publishing from your ongoing research as a work in progress. But there is more. There are considerations of modern or current takes on methodology, method, techniques, strategies, and so on, that suggest themselves. This means that you can offer new insights to older works, classics even, with your takes on them. Current researchers, like you, will be looking not only to such works as those of Guba out of works by Denzin and Lincoln (2000), for example, but also for more recent ones pertaining to current research on such subjects as are discussed in such works.

There are pertinent considerations for new issues being researched (yours, for example), and issues emerging from literature reviews in the area of your research. Other researchers, as well as editors and publishers, are eager for such knowledge as you would be able to provide. There is also what you might have to offer in relation to the research journey itself, such as in relation to supervision from the student perspective, and you have an eager audience just waiting to hear from you. Current researchers need the most recent considerations on classic works and issues. Think of ones that you have grappled with: validity, insider researcher, at risk research subjects, ethics issues, critiques of established methods and techniques ... you could generate quite a list here. After all, at this point in your career as a researcher, you are ideally placed to identify what others need in current literature on research.

Possibilities for writing

Methodology

There are issues of methodology in general as well as methodology in particular to consider. Papers may be generated out of these. If you are working in the poststructuralist area, you have further suggestive possibilities in things like feminist and post-feminist approaches to research, the construction of subjectivities, the mobilization of discourses, modern constructions of regimes of truth, and so on. If you are drawing on phenomenology, you may explore the implications of the concept of lived experience in general terms, and you may go into particulars of van Manen's (1990) posited life-world existentials, or Husserl's (1931) idea of bracketing and how this is done when you employ phenomenology. Who else, after all, is publishing about these things that you have found that you can use? Perhaps you might write a piece examining just how the researcher goes about bracketing, and in doing this go beyond a declaration that it is to be done. If you are going with symbolic interactionism, you may write a piece that focuses on the construction of texts as symbols, or research participants' interaction with texts. And while you're at it, what about a consideration of being participants in research rather than being subjects of it?

Method

Your method chapter offers similarly fertile ground to exploit. Classic works on case study will be major informing works for all researchers employing this method. If you are one of these, you will have come up against particular aspects of this in relation to your own work that may be teased out a little, published, and help to inform the work of others as well. If you are working with ethnography, you may help to advance the thinking in this area by making public how it has affected the ways in which you have conducted your own research.

Discourse analysis is a standard approach to data analysis in poststructuralist work and may be explored alongside document analysis as part of discursive practice and construction of subjectivities. While narrative representations of research outcomes are becoming increasingly visible on the research scene, they are still rare enough and new enough to attract the attention of editors, publishers, and the research audience. Given this, then, there is further scope for your engaging critiques of method(s), many of which have become dated and are probably in need of some stiff critiques themselves (see for example Bourdieu's, 1977, critique of phenomenology) and others which may be in need of some current researcher's support and even argument for relevance (such as the work of Kuhn, 1970).

Techniques

If you are using, or have already used, focus groups you will have read the literature that outlines their advantages and disadvantages, as well as the conditions for their effective use. You may put this together in relation to their influence on your work and extend the literature available on this subject. The same may be done for individual interviews. One that stands out is Thompson's (1996) work on taping and the tape recorder in gathering data. Just as she did, you have the possibility of publishing material on difficulties and how to overcome them (marginalized groups, children, and so on) when collecting data.

Literature review

Writing the literature review for your thesis carries within it the trap of using it to show off all that you have read without referring to ways in which this informs your research design as it addresses a gap in the literature while mapping issues in your field, giving an overview of current debate(s) in the literature, and identifying current and emerging problems. Once you have got past the showing off problem, though, what you have is pure gold for other researchers in your field, should you decide to work it into a publication. They can mine it for literature to consult themselves, and they can see the field as you lay it out for their consideration. It is likely that your literature review will have picked up on conflicting views and representations, with the added benefit of your having positioned these historically as developments in thinking have emerged and been identified by you. Given such an extra dimension, your own writing in that chapter of your thesis can form the substance of a publishable essay.

Ethics

Your consideration of ethics is another chapter of the thesis, and again, suggests scope for publication as you identify ethics issues, and how to deal with them. You will have come up with things like safeguards to ensure that your research does no harm (the key consideration in ethics); you will possibly have come up against and dealt with issues of participant reluctance. Publishing your work on this sort of thing may inform that of others.

Validity

Your considerations of validity will have been of most serious importance in your research, and you will have explained how you have dealt with them in your thesis. Yet what have you found in the literature on validity to inform your work? You will have had to engage your own discussion of concepts and terms in relation to this and argued your way out of quantitative research conventions that tend to overshadow our qualitative research. Think, for a moment...to whom have you turned? Two people stand out in this regard: Lather (1986, 1993) and her concept of trustworthiness, and Scheurich (1997) with his wonderful title of *Masks of Validity* in the conduct of qualitative research. Everybody uses these, because nobody else much has been publishing on this, and they are dated. You might consider putting together a paper around your own discussions on this theme (perhaps including some discussion on bracketing here too).

Research journeys

It never ceases to surprise how popular personal accounts of individual research journeys are, and how often they are published or presented at conferences to appear in conference proceedings. What you base this writing on, as always in research writing, is theory to support your considerations. You may look at the your country's policy and procedures in training its researchers in relation to the Lave and Wenger (1994) concept of Legitimate Peripheral Participation (LPP), or Vygotsky's (1978) concept of the Zone of Proximal Development (ZPD), perhaps extending it to the concept of scaffolding of research undertakings at candidature levels. This would provide a theoretical framework for dealing with problems, identifying hurdles overcome, and managing your supervisor(s)...a more popular and resonant topic among candidates than you might think.

Possibilities for publications

Journals that you have been consulting for your own thesis present as obvious possibilities for publications, as do publishers of books that have been consulting for your own thesis. As you consult these, and get familiar with their Web pages, editorial boards, and mailing lists, you will have opportunities to respond to editors' calls for papers and calls for chapters of books when issues in your field come up. You can submit at any time on any topic regardless of whether you come across such calls or not. When you do hit upon a particular journal for possible publication, though, make sure that you are familiar with it and the readership it serves, so that you do not waste everybody's time by submitting your excellent writing to a journal that does not publish this sort of paper.

Consult the *Advice to Contributors* or *Advice to Authors* on journals' Web pages in the first instance. You may also respond to specific calls for papers or chapters, where the instructions are given. If you are at the stage, usually after successful completion of the degree, where you have a book possibility out of your thesis, complete the publisher's book proposal forms, but when you do, ensure that you have a publications record to help to sell your proposal. Most importantly, don't be discouraged by rejections... try another journal or publisher, but make sure that you take note of feedback on reasons for rejection, and attend to these.

Conclusion

If you are being honest with yourself, you have not strictly kept to a narrowly focussed reading program as you have engaged your own research. You have gone on incredibly interesting but tangential paths, reading widely, and in doing so, have encountered issues that go beyond the focus of your thesis. You have not been able to pursue all of these in your thesis, but now you are able to raise such issues in academic papers, foregrounding interesting perspectives that, while apparently marginal as far as your work is concerned, nevertheless may have a good deal of interest for others working in your field. These you can work into publications.

Publishers and their agents are always on the lookout for good publishing ideas. Remember, you have an advantage because of the uniqueness of your research. That's why you got your university place as a candidate to begin with. Since you started on your own research, you have gained experience in scholarly writing in the development of your own thesis...another advantage. What is more, you are widely read on current issues in your field and current research in general. You know not only what is not there, but also what you needed to have there. If you did, so did others; editors will be very much aware of this as well. They will be acutely aware of what their journals or books have not addressed. It is all stacked in your favor.

Suggested reading

Scholarly articles, book chapters, and books in your field of interest will serve not only to inform you as far as content is concerned, but also in relation to matters of style and approach. There are some texts that focus specifically on this publishing dimension of your work.

Germano, W. (2005) *From dissertation to book* is a particularly detailed and valuable discussion of what is involved in this important endeavor by a PhD graduate.

Susan Rabiner and Alfred Fortunato's (2003) *Thinking like your editor: How to write great serious nonfiction and get it published* has maintained it popularity with readers since its publication, with good practical advice.

Sarah Caro's (2009) *How to publish your PhD* says it all in its title, and takes into account more recent developments in the field. It has the advantage of more current perspectives as it canvasses issues that suggest themselves in relation to new technologies and globalization and their possible influences on modern academic publishing.

There is also advice from publishers themselves, keen to get fresh ideas from knowledgeable scholars (see, e.g., www.tandf.co.uk/journals/authorservices and such like), personal blogs from successful (and otherwise) PhD graduate publishers of their own work, whose stories may be of interest to you. You might even like to post your own.

Hot Tip 12

A rejection of a well-written, scholarly, genre-informed article by the editor of one journal in all probability really means that you have selected the wrong journal. You know that it is a good paper, so submit it to another, more appropriate journal. And then start on your next one.

References

Australian Institute for Aboriginal and Strait Islander Studies. (2012). *Guidelines for ethical research in Aboriginal and Torres Strait Islander studies*. IATSIS. http://www.aiatsis.gov.au/research/ethics/documents/GERAIS.pdf.

Baker, J. (1998). Gender, race and PhD completion in Natural Science and Engineering. *Economics of Education Review*, *17*(2), 179–188.

Bell, J. (1995). *Doing your research project: A guide for first-time researchers in education and social science*. Buckingham: Open University Press.

Blaikie, N. (1993). *Approaches to social enquiry*. Cambridge: Polity.

Blair, T. (2001, 23 May). The prime minister launching Labour's education manifesto at the University of Southampton. From http://www.theguardian.com/politics/2001/may/23/labour.tonyblair.

Block, D. (1995). Social constraints on interviews. *Prospect*, *10*(3), 35–48.

Bloor, M., Frankland, J., Thomas, M., & Robson, K. (2001). *Focus groups in social research*. Thousand Oaks: Sage.

Bourdieu, P. (1977). *Outline of a theory of practice (N. Richard, Trans.)*. Cambridge and New York: Cambridge University Press.

Bruce, C. S. (1994). Research students' early experiences of the dissertation literature review. *Studies in Higher Education*, *19*(2), 217–229.

Bryman, A. (2009). *Social research methods*. Oxford: Oxford University Press.

Bunton, D. (2005). The structure of PhD conclusion chapters. *Journal of English for Academic Purposes*, *4*(3), 207–224.

Caro, S. (2009). *How to publish your PhD*. Oxford: Oxford University Press.

Charon, J. M. (2009). *Symbolic interactionism: An introduction, an interpretation, an integration*. Upper Saddle River, NJ: Prentice Hall.

Cohen, D., Manion, L., & Harrison, K. (2000). *Research methods in education*. London: Routledge.

Cooper, H. M. (1989). *Integrating research: A guide for literature reviews*. Newbury Park: Sage.

Council of Australian Deans and Directors of Graduate Studies. (2005). Guidelines to support the framework for best practice in generic capabilities for research students in Australian universities. http://www.ddogs.edu.au/#mainPage.

Crotty, M. (1998). *The foundations of social research: Meaning and perspective in the research process*. London: Sage.

Denzin, N. (1992). *Symbolic interactionism and cultural studies: The politics of interpretation*. Chichester: John Wiley & Sons Ltd.

Denzin, N. K. & Lincoln, Y. S. (Eds.), (2000). *Handbook of qualitative research*. Thousand Oaks: Sage.

Derrida, J. (1973). *Speech and phenomena*. Evanston: Northwestern University Press.

Doermann, D., Kise, K., & Marinai, S. (2013). International Journal on Document Analysis and Recognition (IJDAR). Springer.

Flick, U. (2007). *Designing qualitative research*. London: Sage.

Flick, U. (2009). *An introduction to qualitative research*. London: Sage.

Foucault, M. (1973). *Discipline and punish*. London: Penguin.

Fry, S. (2013). *QI* Episode 9: Illness. Sydney November 1: Australian Broadcasting Commission.

Germano, W. (2005). *From dissertation to book*. Chicago: University of Chicago Press.

Grbich, C. (2013). *Qualitative data analysis*. London and Other Places: Sage.

Habermas, J. (1979). *Communication and the evolution of society*. London: Heinemann Educational.

Hakim, C. (1987). *Case studies in research design*. New York: Allen & Unwin.

Hamel, J., Dufour, S., & Fortin, D. (1993). *Case study methods*. Thousand Oaks: Sage.

Hart, C. (2001). *Doing a literature search: A comprehensive guide for the social sciences*. Thousand Oaks: Sage.

Hartley, J. (2004). Case study research. In C. Cassell, & G. Symon (Eds.), *Essential guide to qualitative methods in organizational research* (pp. 323–333). London; Thousand Oaks: Sage.

Headland, T. N. (1990). Emics and etics: The insider/outsider debate. In T. N. Headland, K. L. Pike, & M. Harris (Eds.), *Emics and etics: The insider/outsider debate*. Newbury Park, CA: Sage.

Hillyard, S. (2010). *New frontiers in ethnography*. Bingley, UK: Emerald.

Husserl, E. (1931). *Ideas: General introduction to pure phenomenology (W. R. Boyce Gibson, Trans.)*. London: Allen & Unwin.

Kelley, K., Clark, B., Brown, V., & Sitzia, J. (2003). Good practice in the conduct and reporting of survey research. *The International Society for Quality in Health Care*, *15*(3), 261–266.

Kuhn, T. (1970). *The structure of scientific revolutions*. Chicago: University of Chicago Press.

Lather, P. (1986). Issues of validity in openly ideological research: Between a rock and a soft place. *Interchange*, *17*(Winter), 63–84.

Lather, P. (1993). Fertile obsession: Validity after poststructuralism. *The Sociological Quarterly*, *34*(4), 673–693.

Latona, K., & Browne, M. (2001). *Factors associated with completion and retention of Research Higher Degrees*. Report No. 37, Department of Education, Training and Youth Affairs, Higher Education Division, Canberra.

Lave, J., & Wenger, E. (1994). *Situated learning: Legitimate peripheral participation*. New York: Cambridge University Press.

Leonard, W., & Mertova, P. (2007). *Using narrative inquiry as a research method: An introduction to using critical event narrative*. Oxon: Routledge.

Lyotard, J.-F. (1984). *The postmodern condition: A report on knowledge*. Minneapolis: University of Minnesota Press.

Mathews, J. (1989). *Age of democracy: The politics of post-Fordism*. Oxford: Oxford University Press.

Mc Houl, A., & Grace, W. (1993). *A Foucault primer: Discourse, power and the subject*. Carlton: Melbourne University Press.

Organisation for Economic Cooperation and Development. (2002). *OECD Frascati manual* (6th ed.). OECD. http://stats.oecd.org/glossary/detail.asp?ID=192.

Park, C. (2005). New variant PhD: The changing nature of doctorates in the UK. *Journal of Higher Education Policy and Management*, *27*(2), 189–207.

QSR International Pty Ltd. (2013). *NVivo*. http://www.qsrinternational.com/products/productoverview/comparison.htm.

Rabiner, S., & Fortunato, A. (2003). *Thinking like your editor: How to write great serious nonfiction and get it published*. New York: W. W. Norton & Co.

Ridley, D. (2012). *The literature review: A step-by-step guide for students*. Thousand Oaks: Sage.

Scheurich, J. J. (1997). *Research method in the postmodern*. Bristol: Falmer.

Silverman, D. (2003). *Doing qualitative research: A practical handbook*. Thousand Oaks: Sage.

Stake, R. E. (1995). *The art of case study research*. Thousand Oaks, London and New Delhi: Sage.

Survey Monkey. https://www.surveymonkey.com/.

The Shorter Oxford Dictionary. (1973). London: Oxford University Press.

Thompson, D. (1996). The tape recorder as a mediating factor in research. *The Australian Educational Researcher*, *23*(3), 1–12.

van Manen, M. (1990). *Researching lived experience: Human science for an action-sensitive pedagogy*. New York: State University of New York Press.

Vygotsky, L. S. (1978). *Mind in society: The development of higher psychological processes*. USA: Harvard University Press.

Watson, D. (2005). *Watson's dictionary of weasel words*. Sydney: Vintage (Australia).

Weedon, C. (1988). *Feminist practice and post-structuralist theory*. Oxford, UK: Basil Blackwell Ltd.

Wodak, R., & Meyer, M. (2009). *Methods for critical discourse analysis*. London: Sage.

Wolfinger, N. H. (2002). On writing fieldnotes: Collection strategies and background expectancies. *Qualitative Research*, *2*(1), 85–93.

Yin, R. K. (2003). *Application of case study research* (2nd ed.). Thousand Oaks, London and New Delhi: Sage.

Yin, R. K. (2006). Case study methods. In J. Green, G. Camili, & P. Elmore (Eds.), *Handbook of complementary methods in education research* (pp. 111–122). USA: Lawrence Erlbaum for the American Educational Research Association.

Yin, R. K. (2014). *Case study research: Design and methods*. Beverley Hills: Sage.

Zeegers, M. (2013). *Grammar matters*. South Melbourne: Oxford University Press.

Index

Note: Page numbers followed by *f* indicate figures and *b* indicate boxes.

FSC
www.fsc.org
MIX
Papier | Fördert
gute Waldnutzung
FSC® C083411

Kolibri 360 GmbH
Ferdinand-Jühlke-Straße 7
99095 Erfurt, Deutschland
produktsicherheit@kolibri360.de